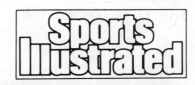

STRENGTH TRAINING

Sports Illustrated Winner's Circle Books

BOOKS ON TEAM SPORTS

Baseball
Basketball
Football: Winning Defense
Football: Winning Offense
Hockey
Lacrosse
Pitching
Soccer

BOOKS ON INDIVIDUAL SPORTS

Bowling
Competitive Swimming
Cross-Country Skiing
Figure Skating
Golf
Racquetball
Running for Women
Skiing
Tennis
Track: Championship Running
Track: The Field Events

SPECIAL BOOKS

Backpacking
Canoeing
Fly Fishing
Scuba Diving
Small-Boat Sailing
Strength Training
Training with Weights

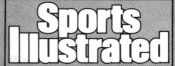

STRENGTH TRAINING

Your Ultimate Weight Conditioning Program

by John Garhammer

Photography by
Heinz Kluetmeier

Sports Illustrated
Winner's Circle Books
New York

Special thanks to Field's Hosiery and Northern Lights Nautilus, both of Burlington, Vt.

Photo credits: Carl Dealoe, p. 46; courtesy of Cybex, Division of Lumex, Inc., p. 54; courtesy of the York Barbell Company, York, Pa., p. 57 (upper right); John Balik, courtesy of Gold's Gym, Venice, Ca., p. 60.

For *Sports Illustrated:* Bill Jaspersohn, pp. 10 (upper right), 75, 162; Walter Iooss, Jr., p. 10 (lower left); Andy Hayt, p. 10 (lower right); Neil Leifer, p. 13 (top); Bruce Klemens, p. 33; Anthony Neste, p. 13 (bottom); Enrico Ferorelli, p. 15; Brian Lanker, p. 174; Jerry Wachter, p. 193.

Drawings on pp. 22 and 25 from *Principles of Anatomy and Physiology,* 4th edition, by Gerard J. Tortora and Nicholas P. Anagnostakos, © 1984 Biological Sciences Textbooks, Inc., A & P Textbooks, Inc., and Elia-Sparta, Inc. Reprinted with permission of Harper & Row, Publishers, Inc. Drawings on p. 24 © Leonard D. Dank.

All diagrams by Kim Llewellyn. All other photographs by Heinz Kluetmeier.

Designer: Kim Llewellyn

Library of Congress Cataloging in Publication Data

Garhammer, John.
  Sports illustrated strength training.

Bibliography: p.
1. Weight lifting. 2. Exercise. I. Sports illustrated (Time, Inc.) II. Title.
GV546.3.G37   1987   613.7′1   87-23491
ISBN 0-452-26041-8 (pbk.)

Contents

Preface

No matter whether you are young or old, male or female, fat or thin, a serious, full-time athlete or an occasional sports participant—this book is for you. It is written to help you improve your physical condition by adding a strength training program to your exercise activities. There are dozens of books in today's marketplace on weight or strength training and other means of exercise for conditioning and fitness. This book differs in several respects, particularly in the approach it takes to prepare you to develop your own productive strength and conditioning program, whatever your final goal. Many strength training books reflect a bias directly related to the authors' own limited background or area of specialization, such as bodybuilding or exercise physiology. Many books present an incomplete picture of weight training. And some books contain a large number of photographs of various exercises but offer little in the way of principles by which the reader can establish or modify an ongoing training program to suit his or her specific goals and needs. In this book I've tried to avoid these shortcomings.

We'll start with an overview of the basic concepts of kinesiology, which is the study of human movement, and exercise physiology, which deals with how the body functions and changes when it's exercised. From there, we'll move to some general properties of a quality strength program and discuss factors to consider when choosing a place to train, including the pros and cons of using some commonly available types of equipment. We'll learn to do a large variety of the most productive strength training exercises, and a series of examples will gradually teach you how to apply basic principles to construct a productive exercise program tailored to your individual needs. Information about good nutrition and its importance to a successful training program is also given; and ergogenic aids—controversial substances such as anabolic steroids that may enhance physical performance—are discussed. In the final chapter you'll find some advanced ideas about combining various types of physical activities in "training cycles." References for additional reading are provided after the last chapter.

My own involvement with strength training began on a Saturday morning in a friend's basement with a typical exercise barbell set. I was 13 years old and found that I could lift 70 pounds, about half my body weight, from the floor to my shoulders and then to arm's length overhead. This result was neither far ahead of nor far behind the abilities of my companions. Having noticed for some time that I was less muscular than some of my friends, I felt—surely influenced somewhat by "muscleman" ads in comic books and sports magazines—that lifting weights would be the great equalizer, if not the means of gaining an edge. As they say, I was bitten by the "iron bug". Soon afterwards, a neighbor and I bought an exercise barbell/dumbbell set from the Sears catalog, and that led to the start of a weight lifting gym in my parents' garage. I've trained with weights constantly ever since and have always been happy with the results. I've also kept a written record of almost every workout over the years and have read everything I could find to gain a better understanding of how to exercise to achieve various goals and why different types of exercise yield different results. This ever-growing interest in strength training and exercise in general eventually led to my doctoral degree in kinesiology at UCLA. This book is an attempt to make many of the most important things I've learned and experienced available to you.

I have covered the topics included in this text in many courses I've taught within the undergraduate, professional, and extension kinesiology programs at the University of California, Los Angeles (UCLA), as well as in courses I've taught at Auburn University and in strength training lectures and clinics I've given at the former U.S. Olympic Training Center in Squaw Valley, at the current Olympic Training Center in Colorado Springs, and at other locations throughout the United States during the past 15 years. I have tried to make the material in this book as up-to-date as possible, and in doing so I have made use of information from numerous sources on the development of functional strength and overall conditioning of the body. I hope and expect that you will find in this book what you need to understand and use strength training to develop a stronger, more powerful, and healthier body.

Though impossible to name all those who have contributed to my involvement in strength training, I would like to acknowledge and thank the following individuals, who added most significantly to my enjoyment and understanding of the "iron game" as either a coach, a scientist, or a fellow athlete: Brian Derwin, Walter Good, Bob Hise, Dave Laut, Carl Miller, John Pat O'Shea, Bill Starr, Mike Stone, Al Treaster, and Dave Wagner.

Special credit is given to Drs. Michael Stone and Ralph Rozenek for technical contributions during preparation of the manuscript.

Very special thanks to Jean Davis, Bob Rich, and Linda Polin for typing, word-processing, and proofreading during various stages of manuscript preparation, and to my parents, who parked their car on the street for several years so that I could have a gym and train in the garage.

Appreciation is extended to Donn Swanbom, Patti Bruckman, Paul Staub, Diane Fuhrman, Heinz Kluetmeier, and Bill Jaspersohn, who contributed a lot of effort and showed great patience during two very long days of shooting the photographs used in this book.

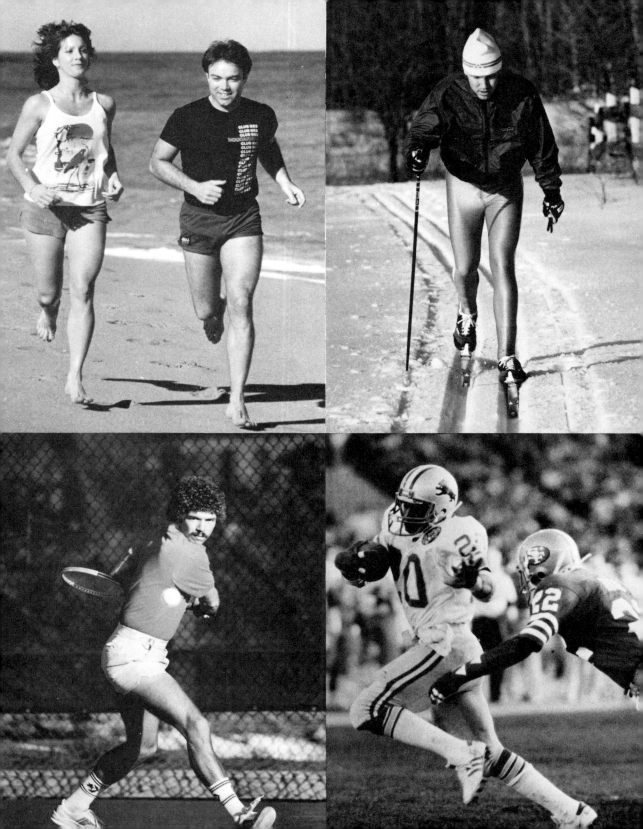

Introduction

In the past decade or two we have seen a worldwide boom of interest in physical fitness—and with good reason: People everywhere have discovered that the pursuit of physical fitness is one of the most rewarding activities in which they can engage. Everyone knows the short-term and long-term benefits of physical fitness for health, vitality, self-image, and the ability to function closer to one's ultimate potential in work and recreation. But not all of us understand that total body fitness is the product of several components. Two of these are *muscular endurance* and *cardiovascular fitness,* as exemplified by the jogging craze. A third is *improved body composition*—that is, reasonable body fat levels. Countless diet plans bear witness to the pursuit of this component. Frequently, however, we overlook *muscular strength, power,* and *joint flexibility* as additional components of total body fitness.

Typical endurance exercise, such as jogging or swimming and cycling longer distances, certainly does enhance muscular endurance for at least some muscle groups, improves cardiovascular fitness, and helps us reduce body fat. But the fact is that strength, power, and flexibility are not, in general, improved, and may even be lowered by

11

No matter who you are or what form of physical activity you pursue, your overall fitness can be improved by some form of strength training.

such activities. Research has shown that to produce improvement in all the components of fitness—muscular endurance, cardiovascular fitness, reasonable body fat levels, muscular strength and power, and joint flexibility—requires an exercise program incorporating some weight lifting or overload training. Usually some combination of weight lifting and endurance exercise (jogging, swimming, rowing, cycling, cross-country skiing) will produce the best results relative to overall fitness. We'll talk about what's right for your exercise program based on your needs in the following chapters.

MISCONCEPTIONS ABOUT STRENGTH TRAINING

Until recent years the extensive benefits possible from strength training received little attention. The reasons were numerous. One was the lack of an acceptable image for weight lifting as exercise. You may be one among many who related lifting weights to big-muscled, sweaty men grunting and groaning as they "pumped iron" in dingy basements and windowless back rooms. Another misconception was the lack of differentiation between weight lifting for exercise and the specialized sports of Olympic weightlifting, powerlifting, and body-building. Let's clear up this misunderstanding right off by discussing these "iron game" sports.

Olympic Weightlifting

Olympic weightlifting is the form of amateur competitive lifting that has been included in the Olympic Games almost continuously since their revival in 1896. The lifting movements contested have changed over the years and since 1972 have included only the "snatch" and "clean and jerk" lifts, which are discussed in Chapter 4. These lifts are characterized by speed of movement, balance, full range of joint movements, explosive strength (power), timing, and total body involvement. Because of these characteristics, Olympic-style lifting is the most athletic of the three sports associated with lifting weights. The first U.S. Women's National Olympic Weightlifting Championship was held in 1981. Many top athletes in other "explosive" sports, such as throwing and jumping events in track and field, use some of the same lifting movements that Olympic weightlifters use in their training. It should be noted that the single word "weightlifting" is the correct term for this sport. The two words "weight lifting"—and the words "weight training"—refer to using weights in an exercise program.

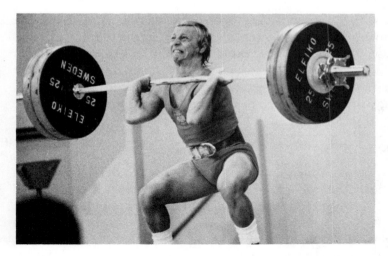

Olympic-style lifting: the most athletic of the three sports associated with lifting weights.

Powerlifting

Powerlifting developed as an amateur competitive sport largely in the United States during the 1960s. The first United States Championship was held in 1965 and the first World Championship in 1972. The lifts now performed in competition are the squat, bench press, and deadlift, which are discussed in Chapter 4. These lifts can be characterized as requiring strength rather than power (that is, strength with fast movement), though the sport's name implies the opposite. The lifts in powerlifting are done much more slowly and involve more limited ranges of joint movement than the Olympic lifts. Yet the use of all or some of these lifts in general strength training is extremely valuable because they de-

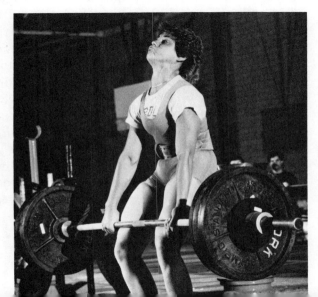

The squat, the bench press, and the dead lift (shown here) are the three exercises performed in competitive powerlifting.

velop the larger muscle groups in the legs, hips, back, chest, and shoulders. The sport itself has grown at an extremely rapid rate since 1965, in the United States and many other countries. Part of the reason is that the lifts are relatively easy to learn and reasonably heavy weights can be lifted without years of extensive training. In recent years, women's participation in powerlifting has grown rapidly, and is now more extensive than women's participation in Olympic lifting.

Bodybuilding

Bodybuilding is an activity in which participants seek the development of a well-defined, muscular, and symmetrical body. Success in competition is based on the subjective opinions of judges as opposed to the more objective criteria of the amount of weight contestants can lift (as in Olympic weightlifting and powerlifting). Bodybuilders often use some basic lifting movements found in powerlifting and, to a lesser extent, Olympic lifting to develop their bodies, in addition to specialized exercises that isolate and develop smaller muscles and muscle groups. Diet is a critical part of a bodybuilder's training program since body fat must be low for success in competition. Women's bodybuilding competitions have become frequent and popular throughout the United States in recent years, and the presence of cash prizes in professional bodybuilding contests in general has contributed to the rapid growth of the sport in the past decade.

A national or international caliber competitor in any of the above three "iron game" sports may or may not possess total fitness. No doubt the individual will be strong, but flexibility will depend on the sport and whether or not the athlete uses stretching in his or her training program. Research has shown that Olympic lifters, for example, have good flexibility. In fact, measurements taken at the 1964 and 1976 Olympic Games indicated that only the gymnasts had better flexibility than the weightlifters. This should make it clear to you that lifting even very heavy weights does not mean you will lose flexibility or become muscle-bound. Power outputs for weightlifters have also been measured as very high. However, endurance, cardiovascular fitness, and body composition may or may not be good for athletes in any of the above "iron game" sports, depending on their overall training programs, other physical activity habits, diet, and genetic traits. *But total fitness need not be sacrificed if you're one who decides to lift weights exclusively.* In later chapters I'll show you ways in which you can attain *total* fitness through a well-designed weight training program with or without additional modes of exercise.

Another important reason for the slow recognition of the benefits of

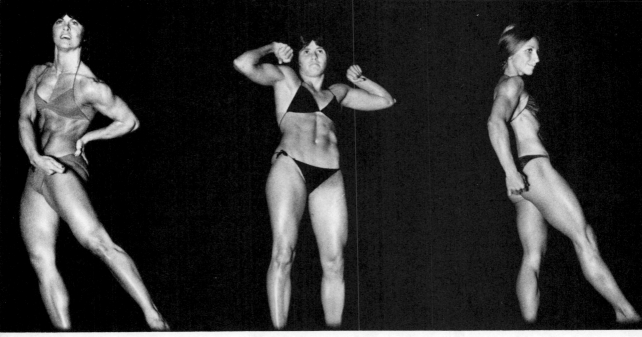

Body builders are usually more interested in muscle definition than in strength.

strength training was the lack of research done to determine and quantify the physiological responses and adaptations of the body to this type of exercise. Early research efforts in strength training were generally very limited in scope and involved resistive exercise programs that were not properly designed and balanced. They emphasized the single goal of increasing the maximum weight a person could lift, once, in a few basic lifting movements (the so-called one repetition max, or 1 RM measurement).

Today we have a better understanding of the variety of benefits possible from strength training. The notion that anyone—not just an athlete or a body-builder—can profit from lifting weights is becoming more and more accepted. As a result, we have witnessed an incredible growth of health spas and exercise gyms featuring a variety of weight lifting equipment. Sales of weight equipment for home use have soared. Increasing numbers of people and sports teams at all levels are including strength training in their pursuit of total fitness and improved athletic performance.

The goal of the following chapters is to provide you with information, based on research and empirical findings, about the functioning of the body and the effects on it of various types of exercise. After that, I'll show you how you can structure both short-term and long-term training programs to achieve your goals in physical fitness and better performance.

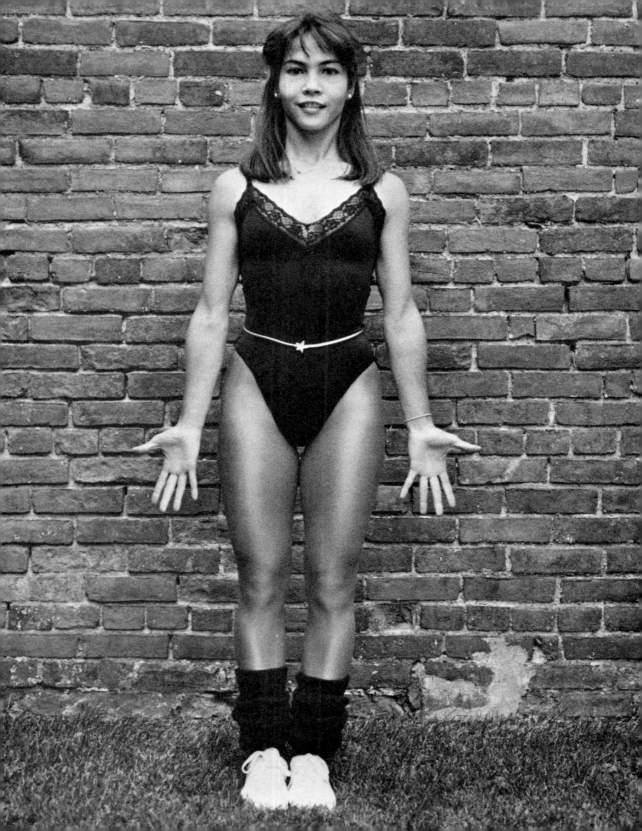

1

The Basic Kinesiology of Exercise: How Our Bodies Move

You don't have to be an expert, but to understand how to exercise for strength fitness, you do need some insights into the basic functioning of your body.

The bones making up your skeletal system are connected at joints that permit a variety of movements when muscles crossing these joints contract. We'll first consider the primary movements possible at your body's major joints, such as the knee, elbow, or shoulder; the muscles that control each joint's movements; and the proper terminology to describe these movements accurately. You'll find that once you understand how your joints move and how your muscles contract to produce various joint movements, you'll have a better appreciation of the processes occurring when you lift weights.

MOVEMENT TERMINOLOGY

To talk about movements at the various joints, we first position the body in what is known in kinesiology as the *anatomical reference position,* as shown in the photograph at the beginning of this chapter. In this upright standing position, the

17

The anatomical reference position (shown here) is used by kinesiologists to describe various movements of the human body.

arms are held at the side and the palms face forward. Incidentally, the movement terms introduced below are often used in the names of actual strength training exercises. For example, the most common front or back movement of a body part from the reference position is called a *flexion*, and the return of the body part from its flexed position along its original path of motion is called an *extension* (one of the first exercises we'll learn in Chapter 4 is the "knee extension"). When an extension motion continues past the anatomical reference position, the moving joint is said to *hyperextend*. Some joints, such as those in the neck and spine, can hyperextend through a considerable range of motion. Others, such as the hip and shoulder joints, have more limited ranges of hyperextension, while still others such as the knee and elbow do not normally hyperextend without injury. When performing weight lifting exercises, it's almost always desirable to move the joints involved through the full normal range of motion. This helps maintain or improve flexibility and reduce any risk of injury.

Another group of movements involve motion of a body part sideways. Relative to the same reference position, any sideward movement of a limb away from the midline of the body is called an *abduction* at the moving joint. Spreading your fingers and toes apart is referred to in kinesiology as abduction

Examples of Movement Terminology
(A) Flexion (of the hip joint). (B) Extension (of the shoulder) from a flexed position. (C) Hyperextension (of neck and spinal column). (D) Abduction (of both shoulder joints

A   B   C

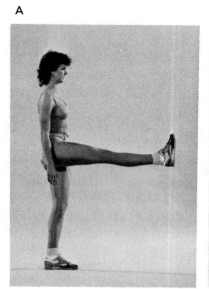 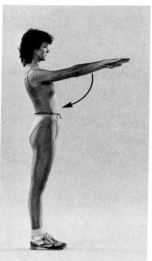 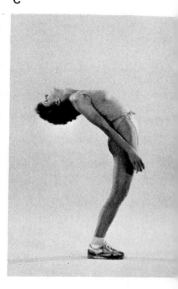

of these segments; lifting a dumbbell sideways away from your body with a straight arm involves abduction at the shoulder. Joints such as the elbow and knee do not normally permit abduction without injury. Return of an abducted limb, along the same path of motion toward the reference position, is called *adduction* at the moving joint. The neck and torso can also tilt sideways to the right or left, and these movements are called *lateral flexions*.

Twisting or *rotational movements* are also common at many joints. The neck and torso can rotate to the right or left, while the shoulder and hip can rotate inward or outward (medially or laterally in kinesiological terms). Some joints, such as the elbow, do not permit rotation without injury. Notice, however, that you can rotate your hand so that your palm faces either toward you or away from you. This is possible due to unique movements of bones in your forearm. These movements are called pronation (palm facing backward) and supination (palm facing as it is in the anatomical reference position). Although a number of other movements or combinations of movements can be defined, those covered above include the majority that you will perform in weight lifting exercises, as well as in normal daily activities. A few less common movement terms will be introduced later in this chapter.

and the right hip joint). (E) Adduction (of the right shoulder) from an abducted position. (F) Lateral flexion (of the spine). (G) Rotation right (of the neck and spine).

D

E

F

G

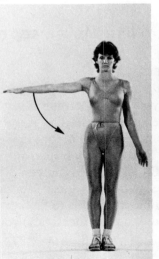
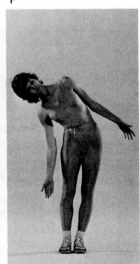
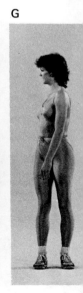

MUSCLES THAT CONTROL MOVEMENT

One of the reasons individual joints move as they do is the way they're structured. The elbow, for example, is a *hinge joint* and permits only flexion and extension—just as a door hinge permits a door to rotate open or closed—about only one axis. The shoulder and hip, by contrast, are *ball and socket joints* and permit movement in virtually all directions. A muscle's position in the body and how its attachment crosses a joint also determines how that joint moves. Muscles attach to bones via tendons and, with few exceptions, have attachments that span one or two joints. Ligaments help hold bones together at joints but, unlike muscles, can't contract.

To discuss all of the muscles of the body is beyond the scope of a book on strength training. However, to help you understand how your body moves as you exercise, you should be familiar with major muscle groups and representative muscles that control movements at the major joints. As you read about the various muscles below, refer to the bone and muscle charts presented on pages 28 and 144–45.

Kinesiologists have a simple set of terms for describing areas of the body's parts. The term *anterior* indicates the front surface of a body segment; *posterior* indicates the rear surface; *lateral* indicates the surface of a body part facing away from the body's midline; and *medial* indicates the surface of a body part facing toward the body's midline. For example, *anterior torso* means the chest and abdomen, *posterior torso* means the upper and lower back, *lateral side of the thigh* means the side facing away from the body, and *medial side of the thigh* means the side facing the opposite leg.

Muscles Controlling Movement at the Ankle Joint

The Tibialis Anterior

While seated or balanced on the opposite foot, lift the toes and the ball of your foot. The muscle you feel tightening along the outside (lateral) edge of your shin, just below the kneecap (patella), is the *tibialis anterior*. This long, narrow muscle plays an important role in foot movement and placement during walking and running. The forefoot lifting motion you performed is called *dorsi flexion* of the ankle joint, and you can strengthen your tibialis anterior by applying resistance to the top (dorsal) surface of your foot near the toes while dorsi flexing. A simple method is to lie face down on a mattress with your feet just over the edge and to push (dorsi flex) your toes into the mattress side. After

ten or twenty repetitions, depending on how much you've used your tibialis
anterior in the past, it will have had a pretty fair workout.

The Soleus and Gastrocnemius

When you lift your heels off the ground and rise on your toes you perform a
movement at the ankle joint called *plantar flexion.* The two muscles that form
the "calf" on the posterior side of your lower leg control this motion. These
two muscles, the *soleus* and *gastrocnemius,* are utilized differently depending
on how fast you move your foot. The reason for this involves the muscle fiber
composition of each muscle (more on muscle fibers later in this chapter). You
can strengthen your calf muscles by rising repeatedly on your toes, perhaps
adding some sort of load on your shoulders for extra resistance.

Muscles Controlling Movement at the Knee Joint

The "Quadriceps"

The knee joint must support all the body weight above it during many complex
movements. Fortunately, tendons of the muscles that control flexion and extension at the knee joint cross the front and back of the knee and aid many
ligaments in stabilizing the joint. This type of added "muscle" support is found
at most of our bone junctions. The four *"quadricep"* muscles—the *rectus
femoris, vastus lateralis, vastus medialis,* and *vastus intermedius*—control *knee
extension* and form the anterior portion of the thigh. You can strengthen your
"quads" by rising repeatedly from a squatting position with or without resistance added to your body weight.

The "Hamstrings"

Three muscles located in the posterior thigh and commonly called the hamstrings control *knee flexion;* they are the *biceps femoris,* the *semitendinosus,*
and the *semimembranosus.* Strengthening the "hams" can help you avoid
hamstring pulls when you run fast, and can most easily be accomplished with
a "leg curl" bench, which permits knee flexion with added resistance.

Muscles Controlling Movement at the Hip Joint

The Rectus Femoris and Iliopsoas Muscle Group

As mentioned earlier, the ball and socket nature of the hip joint permits
movement in virtually all directions. Flexion of the hip is controlled by several

muscles, but we need only concern ourselves with a couple of representative "prime movers." We noted earlier that the *rectus femoris* is a knee extensor; it is also the only member of the quadricep muscle group to cross the hip joint and aid in *hip flexion*. The lesser known *iliopsoas group (iliacus* and *psoas)* is another important contributor to *hip flexion*. These muscles are located deep within our lower abdominal cavity, as shown in the illustration. Note that the psoas originates from the lower lumbar region of the spine; this is important to remember when we discuss abdominal exercises in Chapter 4. Any activity requiring high and forceful thigh lift, such as running up stairs, will develop these and the other hip flexors.

Location of the Iliopsoas Muscle Group

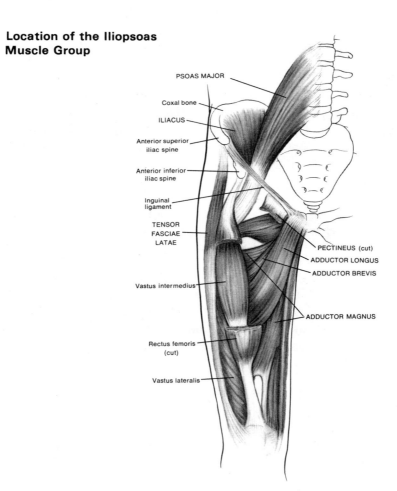

PSOAS MAJOR

Coxal bone

ILIACUS

Anterior superior iliac spine

Anterior inferior iliac spine

Inguinal ligament

TENSOR FASCIAE LATAE

Vastus intermedius

Rectus femoris (cut)

Vastus lateralis

PECTINEUS (cut)

ADDUCTOR LONGUS

ADDUCTOR BREVIS

ADDUCTOR MAGNUS

The Gluteals and Other Hip Muscles

The hamstrings, which flex the knee, are "two-joint" muscles which also cross behind the hip joint and control *hip extension* and *hyperextension.* When you are running fast, your thigh rapidly extends while your knee flexes. Since both these movements are controlled by the hamstrings, people who place a premium on running fast, such as sprinters and running backs in football, commonly suffer from pulled (strained) hamstring muscles. The familiar *gluteus maximus* is the largest of the three gluteal muscles that form the buttocks. It's a very powerful *hip extensor,* while the two smaller gluteals *(medius* and *minimus)* control *hip abduction.* As with the quadriceps, you can develop your gluteals with various deep knee bend (squatting) exercises. Keep in mind that the gluteus maximus is used only in forceful hip extension movements (such as when a ballet dancer jumps) and when the range of motion is great. Simple walking or slow jogging activities do not activate the gluteus maximus, whereas climbing stairs, sprinting, and most weight training exercises involving hip extension do. *Hip adduction* is controlled by the *adductor group—magnus, longeus,* and *brevis*—located in the upper medial part of the thigh. You can strengthen these muscles by adducting your leg with a pulley cable attached to your foot or ankle so as to lift an adjustable resistance, or a training partner can manually resist your attempt at adducting your legs.

Muscles Controlling Movement of the Spinal Column

The Abdominal and Spinal Erector Muscles

To understand the movements of the spinal column it is important to think of it in terms of an upper (cervical), a middle (thoracic), and a lower (lumbar) part. The bones (vertebrae) making up each part are structured somewhat differently, and these differences determine the various bending and rotation movements possible from section to section along the spinal column. The lowest lumbar vertebra rests on the sacrum, which also joins the right and left half of the pelvis. Our ability to *extend, hyperextend,* and *laterally flex* our spinal column is largely dependent on a group of many muscles called the *spinal erectors.* They run up the back from the pelvis and sacrum on both sides of the spinal column and attach to various vertebrae and posterior rib surfaces. The ribs are joined to the middle (thoracic) vertebrae in the back and to the breastbone (sternum) in the front. The natural upward pull of the spinal erectors on the pelvis tends to balance the natural downward pull of hip extensor muscles, such as the hamstrings, which also attach to the posterior pelvis. The *abdominal muscles*

The Skeletal System of the Human Body

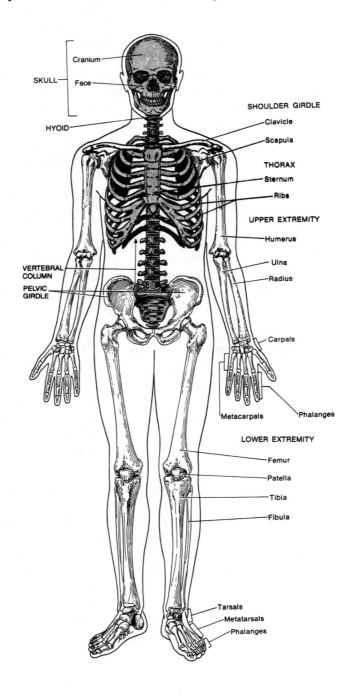

Muscle Locations on the Anterior (Front) and Posterior (Back) Surfaces of the Human Body

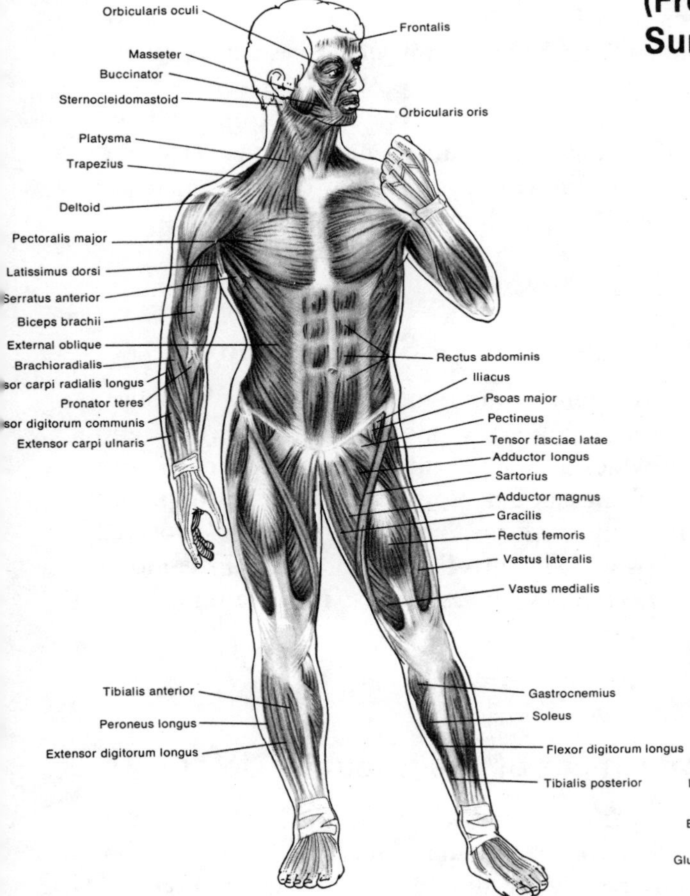

Anterior (Front)

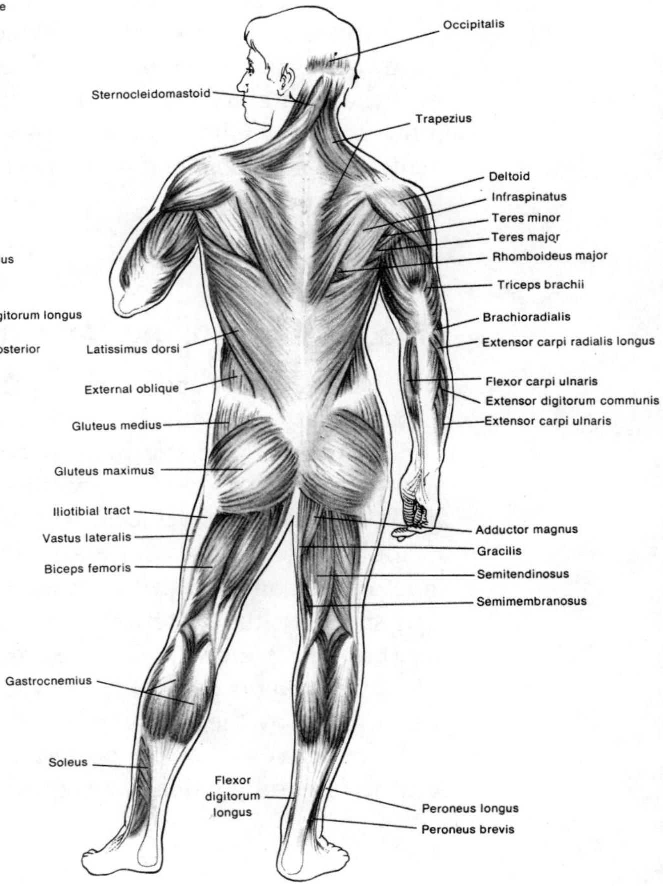

- Orbicularis oculi
- Frontalis
- Masseter
- Buccinator
- Sternocleidomastoid
- Orbicularis oris
- Platysma
- Trapezius
- Deltoid
- Pectoralis major
- Latissimus dorsi
- Serratus anterior
- Biceps brachii
- External oblique
- Brachioradialis
- sor carpi radialis longus
- Pronator teres
- sor digitorum communis
- Extensor carpi ulnaris
- Rectus abdominis
- Iliacus
- Psoas major
- Pectineus
- Tensor fasciae latae
- Adductor longus
- Sartorius
- Adductor magnus
- Gracilis
- Rectus femoris
- Vastus lateralis
- Vastus medialis
- Tibialis anterior
- Peroneus longus
- Extensor digitorum longus
- Gastrocnemius
- Soleus
- Flexor digitorum longus
- Tibialis posterior

Posterior (Back)

- Occipitalis
- Sternocleidomastoid
- Trapezius
- Deltoid
- Infraspinatus
- Teres minor
- Teres major
- Rhomboideus major
- Triceps brachii
- Brachioradialis
- Extensor carpi radialis longus
- Flexor carpi ulnaris
- Extensor digitorum communis
- Extensor carpi ulnaris
- Latissimus dorsi
- External oblique
- Gluteus medius
- Gluteus maximus
- Iliotibial tract
- Vastus lateralis
- Biceps femoris
- Adductor magnus
- Gracilis
- Semitendinosus
- Semimembranosus
- Gastrocnemius
- Soleus
- Flexor digitorum longus
- Peroneus longus
- Peroneus brevis

(rectus abdominis and *internal* and *external obliques)* run from the front of the pelvis upward to anterior rib surfaces and the sternum. Upward pull of the abdominals on the pelvis tends to balance the downward pull of hip flexor muscles, such as the rectus femoris. These various muscle forces acting on our pelvis help us maintain a level pelvis and correct posture. The abdominals control spinal flexion, with the lateral parts *(obliques)* important in rotational and lateral flexion movements of the torso. You can strengthen your "abs" and "erectors" with a variety of exercises, but before you try any of them, there are several factors you should be aware of, which are covered in Chapter 4.

Muscles Controlling Movement of the Shoulder Girdle

The shoulder girdle consists of four bones—the right and left clavicle (collarbone) and scapula (shoulderblade), which are supported on the sternum and upper rib cage. Each scapula provides a "socket" for the shoulder joints, and the upward gliding capability of the shoulder girdle as a whole improves overhead lifting movements involving the arms. The *trapezius muscle* located in the upper back has four sections which control many shoulder girdle movements. The *rhomboid and pectoralis minor muscles* are also important in shoulder girdle movement.

Muscles Controlling Movement of the Shoulder Joint

The rounded upper end of the upper arm bone, known as the humerus, forms a "ball" that joins with the "socket" of the scapula to form the shoulder joint. The large *deltoid muscle* literally covers the shoulder joint, and its three sections—anterior, middle, and posterior—contribute individually or together to all shoulder joint movements. When you raise your arm to the side, as during a shoulder abduction, your entire deltoid is active. If you flex your arm at the shoulder, the anterior deltoid is active. If you forcefully extend or hyperextend your shoulder, the posterior deltoid is used. *Horizontal abduction* at the shoulder (bringing your straight arm from a flexed position in front of you to the side, by moving it parallel to the ground so it finishes in an abducted position) is controlled by the *latissimus dorsi muscle,* located in the upper lateral parts of the back, as well as the posterior deltoid. Any activity where you use your arms to forcefully pull an object toward your body, such as rowing a boat, will develop these muscles. *Horizontal adduction* of the shoulder joint (the opposite of horizontal abduction) is controlled by the *pectoralis major* as well as the anterior deltoid. The "pec" is the large muscle covering each side of the upper anterior torso to form the chest. Any activity where you use your arms to push an object away from your body, such as push-ups, will develop these muscles. Both the pectoralis major and latissimus dorsi contribute to shoulder adduction.

The Smaller Muscles of the Shoulder Joint—The Rotator Cuff

During the many additional complex movements of the shoulder joint, the deltoid, the pectoralis major, and the latissimus dorsi function with other smaller muscles crossing this joint to control motion. Four very important smaller muscles involved in shoulder movements are referred to as the "rotator cuff" muscles *(supraspinatus, infraspinatus, subscapularis,* and *teres minor),* often in the news when injured by a major league pitcher. Members of this muscle group contribute to either internal (medial) or external (lateral) rotation of the shoulder joint, as the name implies. In addition, the tendons of these muscles cross the joint, whether above or from the front or back. These tendons join and surround the head of the humerus, pulling it into the socket of the scapula to help stabilize the joint. Many shoulder injuries involve damage to one or more of the rotator cuff muscles. You'll find a useful exercise for rehabilitating the rotator cuff as well as strengthening the deltoid in Chapter 4 (the lateral raise).

Muscles Controlling Movement at the Elbow Joint

The hinge structure of the elbow joint permits only flexion-extension movements. *Flexion* is controlled by four "flexor" muscles, with the *biceps brachii* (or just biceps), located on the anterior surface of the upper arm, being the most familiar. Elbow *extension* is controlled primarily by the large *triceps brachii* (or just triceps), located on the posterior surface of the upper arm. Any movement requiring forceful extension at the elbow will develop your triceps, while any forceful flexion at the elbow will develop your four elbow flexors.

Muscles Controlling Movement of the Wrist and Hand

Muscles controlling wrist, hand, and finger movements are located primarily in the forearm and have long tendons crossing the wrist and finger joints. Because of the large variety of possible movements and the many controlling muscles, it is easiest to think of these muscles as either *wrist and finger flexors* or *extensors*. Flexors tend to be located in the anterior forearm, relative to the anatomical reference position, while extensors are generally found in the posterior forearm.

PRIME MOVERS FOR BASIC JOINT MOVEMENTS

Joint	Movement	Prime Mover
Ankle	Dorsi flexion	Tibialis anterior
	Plantar flexion	Soleus, gastrocnemius
Knee	Flexion	Hamstrings
	Extension	Quadriceps
Hip	Flexion	Rectus femoris, iliopsoas
	Hyperextension, extension	Gluteus maximus, hamstrings
	Abduction	Gluteus medius, minimus
	Adduction	Adductors
	Horizontal abduction	Gluteus medius, minimus
	Horizontal adduction	Adductors
Intervertebral	Flexion	Abdominals
	Hyperextension, extension	Spinal erectors
	Lateral flexion	Spinal erectors, oblique abdominals
	Rotations	Oblique abdominals
Shoulder girdle	Upward glide	Trapezius
Shoulder	Flexion	Anterior deltoid
	Hyperextension, extension	Posterior deltoid
	Abduction	Deltoid
	Adduction	Latissimus dorsi, pectoralis major
	Horizontal abduction	Latissimus dorsi, posterior deltoid
	Horizontal adduction	Pectoralis major, anterior deltoid
Elbow	Flexion	Biceps
	Extension	Triceps
Wrist and fingers	Flexion	Flexors
	Extension	Extensors

Whenever you move part of your body, you can generally consider one or more muscles as *prime movers:* that is, muscles of primary importance in producing the movement. Other muscles may assist the prime movers and are called *synergists,* while still others may help stabilize the joint during the movement. Joints with high mobility, such as the shoulder joint, are less stable than joints with very restricted motion capabilities, such as the elbow, and are very dependent on *stabilizing muscles* to help prevent dislocations. All the muscles we discussed above are prime movers for many common joint motions of your body but may at times act as synergists or stabilizers. They are the muscles we will concentrate on developing in your strength training program. Now, before hearing about some basic principles to use in putting your program together, it's important to understand a few things about the structure of muscles, how they contract when doing work like weight lifting, and how your central nervous system controls those contractions.

MUSCLE STRUCTURE, ENERGY DEVELOPMENT, AND CONTROL

Fast and Slow Twitch Muscle Fibers

Each muscle in your body is composed of many individual muscle cells called *muscle fibers.* These may run longitudinally the entire length of the muscle and join tendons at each end, or may run diagonally for short distances relative to the muscle's total length and join connective tissue strands that eventually connect to tendons. Scientists call the particular arrangement of fibers within a muscle *muscle architecture,* and it has a major effect on the way the whole muscle contracts—on how much force it can generate, how much it shortens during contraction, and even how it is used during different activities.

Fiber type is also important in determining how a muscle performs. The individual fibers in a muscle may be classified as either *fast twitch* (white muscle) or *slow twitch* (red muscle). Fast fibers can generate a large tension rapidly but fatigue quickly. Slow fibers generate a lower maximum tension at a slower rate but do not fatigue easily. These "contractile properties" determine to some extent the types of muscular activity that each type of fiber contributes to. Some of your muscles may contain a large percentage of fast twitch fibers, while the same muscles in your training partner may contain mostly slow twitch fibers. Sprinting and jumping require large forces to be developed rapidly but only for short periods of time, so if you have mostly fast twitch fibers in your leg muscles you should have an advantage in these events. By contrast, distance running or swimming requires smaller forces to be developed less rapidly but continually for long periods. If you have mostly slow twitch fibers in the right muscles you'll probably excel in these types of sports. As a practical example that affects all of us, I'll point out that the soleus of the calf is composed mostly of slow fibers and is important in walking and jogging. The gastrocnemius of the calf has a larger percentage of fast fibers and is important in sprinting and jumping.

Slow fibers can generate energy efficiently when oxygen is available: They contain specialized molecular components that give them their red color and are important for the use of oxygen in metabolizing blood sugar (glucose) and fats to produce energy. The term "aerobic" exercise refers to physical activity of lower intensity and longer duration that depends primarily on the use of oxygen to generate energy (oxidative metabolism), as happens in "aerobic dance." High intensity exercise, such as sprinting, is primarily dependent on energy generated using blood sugar but without oxygen, resulting in the production of lactic acid, and is called "anaerobic" exercise. Fast fibers function well using this non-oxidative (anaerobic) metabolism. At the instant physical activity starts, or increases in intensity, your muscles need energy to contract. This "immediate need" energy comes from energy storage molecules called ATP, which are found in both fast and slow muscle fibers.

It's important for you to know that as you exercise regularly over a period of weeks, months, and years, your muscle fibers adapt or change differently depending on exactly how you train your body. This is related to the "specificity of exercise" principle, which I'll say more about in Chapter 5. It means, for example, that if you exercise primarily at fast, high force activities, such as sprinting and jumping or explosive weight lifting movements, your fast fibers will change in a way that will permit you to perform better at these types of activities. If you train primarily at slower, lower force, longer duration activities, such as jogging, cycling and swimming long distances, or lifting lighter weights slowly for many repetitions (20 or more), your slow fibers will adapt to make you better at these "endurance" oriented events.

You may find the following example from the animal kingdom of interest. Ducks, which fly long distances at relatively slow speeds, have "red meat" for breast muscles, while chickens, which can fly but a few feet, have "white meat"

BASIC PROPERTIES OF FAST AND SLOW MUSCLE FIBERS

Property	Fast Fiber	Slow Fiber
Contraction time	Fast	Slow
Peak tension	High	Low
Endurance	Very little	Very great
Oxidative capacity	Low	High
Blood supply	Low	High
Mitochondria*	Few	Many
ATPase†	High	Low
Fiber diameter	Large	Small

*Specialized units within muscle cells that utilize oxygen to produce energy-carrying molecules (ATP).
†Enzyme important for rapid muscle contraction.

POSSIBLE ADAPTATIONS OF FAST AND SLOW MUSCLE FIBERS TO TWO TYPES OF EXERCISE

Strength-Power Exercise	Fiber Type	Endurance Exercise
1. Muscle enlargement (hypertrophy) due to increased contractile proteins	Fast	1. Decreased size
2. Increased storage of ATP	Fast	2. Slower contraction speed
3. Increased levels of non-oxidative enzymes	Fast	3. Lower maximum tension
4. Increased recruitment	Fast	4. Increased levels of oxidative enzymes
5. Stimulation pattern changes		5. Increased capillary blood supply
		6. Increased endurance
1. Decreased levels of oxidative enzymes	Slow	1. Increased size and number of mitochondria
2. Decreased endurance	Slow	2. Increased levels of oxidative enzymes
3. Increased maximum tension	Slow	3. Increased capillary blood supply
4. Higher contraction speed		4. Increased glycogen storage
		5. Increased ability to metabolize fats

for breast muscles. You can probably think of other examples of "light" and "dark" meat in animals that relate to fast and slow muscle fibers and their contraction properties.

The Role of the Nervous System in Controlling Muscle Tension

Typical large muscles in your body contain many thousands of muscle fibers of each type. In order to control the tension when a muscle contracts, the fibers are grouped into *"motor units,"* each consisting of a *motor nerve cell,* located in the spinal cord, and several hundred to well over a thousand muscle fibers. Very small muscles, such as those controlling eye movement, may contain far fewer than a hundred motor units, each of which may consist of 10 to 20 fibers. Each muscle fiber is connected to only one motor nerve, and all fibers of a given motor unit are either of the fast or slow variety. As the need for a given muscle to produce *tension increases,* as when you are trying to lift heavier and heavier weights, the central nervous system may simply *recruit more and more of the available motor units* composing the muscle. Scientists believe that in most situations the central nervous system follows a "size principle" in recruitment order, with smaller, slow motor units called on first and larger, fast motor units last. It is unlikely that all the motor units composing a muscle are ever recruited simultaneously due to the central nervous system's built-in protective inhibitory mechanisms. However, the amazing feats of strength performed by individuals in highly aroused emotional states, or under the influence of drugs, may be explained in part as near-total motor unit recruitment made possible by an overriding of normal inhibitory safeguards.

Besides being able to recruit more motor units to satisfy the requirements of a given muscular task, the nervous system can increase the tension produced by any motor unit by stimulating the controlling motor nerve to fire more frequently in a given time period. Basically, a motor nerve transmits electrochemical signals to its muscle fibers, causing them to contract. An active *motor unit,* for example, may have its *firing rate* increased from 40 to 50 times per second, resulting in a substantial increase in the tension being produced. If the rate a motor nerve fires increases for only an instant before returning to its initial firing rate, the tension output will increase due to the change in firing "pattern." If more and more motor units are activated at the same instant, we say the firing is more *synchronous,* resulting in increased tension.

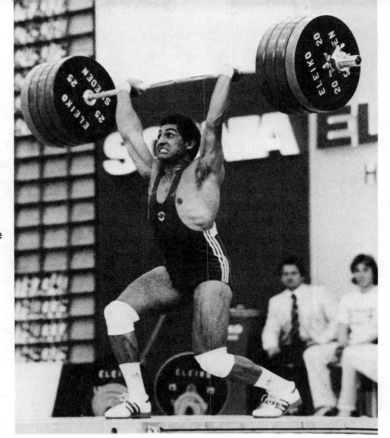

As this world-class lifter shows, you don't necessarily need to develop large muscles to be strong.

In terms of your own strength training, this means that *you don't necessarily have to develop large muscles* (muscle hypertrophy) *to become significantly stronger.* Nervous system control of muscle contraction has a major effect on the tension generated. You can train your nervous system with strength exercises just as you can teach it to learn complex movement skills. Just making regular efforts to lift heavier and heavier weights gradually over weeks and months will produce this desirable training effect.

Hard to believe? Well, the concept is supported by solid scientific evidence, and there are tangible examples of the nervous system's role in increasing strength. One example is found in competitive weightlifters who have been world champions over a period of five to ten years within the same bodyweight class. Since they were highly skilled in lifting technique and maintained low levels of body fat over this span of years, a major part of their ability to lift more weight each year can be attributed to a learning effect within their nervous systems.

TYPES OF MUSCLE CONTRACTION

As you do any exercise you should keep in mind that muscles can produce tension both when they shorten and when they lengthen. The shortening of a muscle is known in strength training and physiology as a *concentric contraction,* whereas the lengthening of a muscle (when its tension is overcome by an external force) is called an *eccentric contraction.* You know an inactive muscle will lengthen when its so-called *"antagonist"* muscle shortens. For example, the bicep (a flexor) at your bent elbow will lengthen when the tricep (an extensor) contracts to straighten your arm. A lengthening or eccentric contraction is different. One would occur, for example, in your shoulder and arm muscles when you attempt too many pull-ups on a chinning bar. As fatigue sets in, these muscles try to shorten (concentric contraction), but the pull of gravity on your body's weight overcomes the muscles' forces and causes them slowly to lengthen. The tricep is not involved in lengthening the bicep in this situation. Between concentric and eccentric contraction, the case of zero contraction velocity occurs; that is, the muscles at a joint neither lengthen nor shorten— there is no movement. In this case, as tension is generated within a muscle, external forces prevent any movement and an *isometric* (constant length) contraction results. Isometric exercises were very popular about 20 years ago. A strength trainee would lock hands together and push or pull as hard as possible to strengthen the pecs, deltoids, or upper back muscles. Busy executives would perform occasional isometric exercises using their desks and feel they were getting a mini-workout. Do isometrics work? Yes and no. They can strengthen some muscles in the joint positions in which the exercises are performed, but not throughout the full range of joint motion that can occur in real-life activities. For complete and truly functional strength increases it's best (with few exceptions) to perform weight lifting exercises that involve multiple joint actions through the fullest possible range of motion.

Keep in mind as you train yourself and gradually get stronger that your physical strength is also related to a number of additional "physiological" factors. These include (1) the length of a muscle at any given point in its range of motion—called the "length-tension" relationship—due to changing amounts of overlap between the thick and thin molecular filaments that make up muscle fibers, and (2) the speed at which a muscle is lengthened or shortened—called the "force-velocity" relationship. Bone lengths and muscle attachment points —so-called leverage factors—also influence how much weight you can lift in various exercises. I'll say a little bit more about some of these factors when we talk about training with weight machines in Chapter 3. But rest assured: No matter what your body type or age, a few weeks on a good strength program will yield results. I know a young woman, for example, who felt extremely uncomfortable doing one or two squats with 50 pounds in her first weight workout, at age 30. A few weeks later she was doing several sets of 10 repetitions in the squat with the same weight. Several months later she was doing 120 pounds for reps in the same exercise. But don't worry about comparing yourself to others (this is a real problem with athletes in their strength programs). The important thing is to make progress for yourself, no matter how fast or slow.

Now let's move on to the principles that can make yours a quality strength training program.

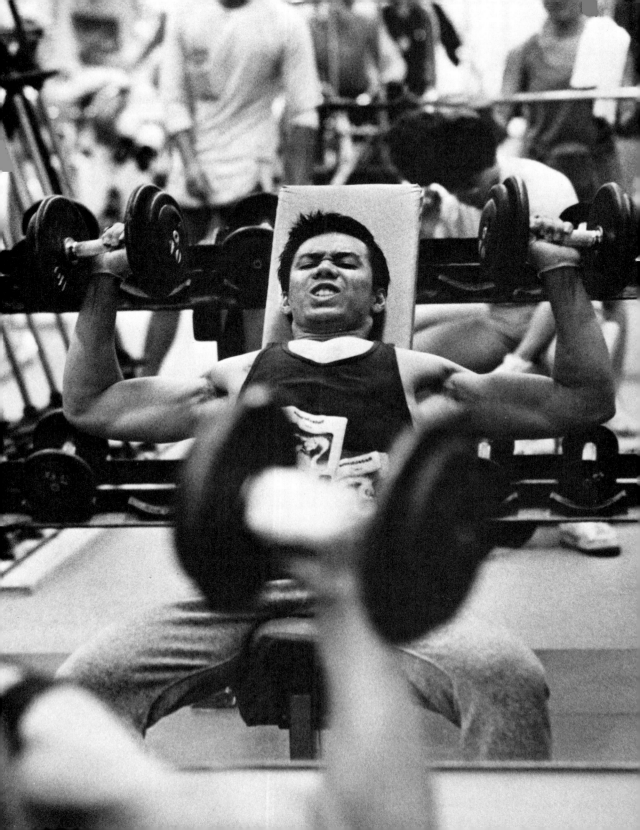

2
Properties of a Quality Strength and Conditioning Program

A quality strength and conditioning program has five characteristics:

1. *All workout sessions begin with a minimum of 10 minutes devoted to general "warm-up" exercises and stretching.* General warm-up refers to such activities as calisthenics, jumping rope, and jogging, which are active in nature. Passive methods of warm-up, such as massage and heat rubs, may be of value in some situations, but active warm-up is usually more important. Indications are that warming up has a positive effect on most types of physical activity and may help to reduce injury potential. The physiological effects of warming up help explain its value. For example, increased muscle temperature results in increased contractile force and speed, while increased blood temperature and flow rate result in increased oxygen delivery to working muscles. A major benefit of warming up is to reduce the likelihood of cardiac ischemia (insufficient blood supply to the heart) during the start of exercise. Experiments have shown that firemen exhibit irregular heartbeats if they go from resting to immediate running, as occurs during work situations. The psychological effect of making a gradual rather than an immediate transition from rest to strenuous

37

The severity of your strength program should match your physical and mental capacities.

physical activity may be another major benefit of warming up.

Part of the overall warm-up process should be devoted to stretching, which aids in developing and maintaining flexibility. Flexibility refers to the range of single and multiple joint motions possible and the ease with which full range movements can be performed. It was once thought that strength-oriented exercises would limit or reduce flexibility, but this has been proven false if weight lifting exercises are performed properly through the entire movement range possible whenever safe to do so.

One important instance when you should limit your movement range slightly is when performing the squat or deep knee bend exercise. The recommended procedure is to squat slowly downward until the thighs are parallel to the ground, and then return to the starting position. Most individuals could squat lower, with more knee flexion, but I discourage this due to the large physical stresses that squatting lower generates at the knee joint. Knee flexibility is usually not a problem and squats will not reduce it, especially when intelligently selected stretching exercises are practiced regularly. The vast majority of lifting exercises can be executed safely using the fullest possible range of motion.

Flexibility may be a contributing factor to reduced injury potential. When

Seven Basic Warm-up Stretches

The shoulder
stretch

The shoulder-girdle
stretch

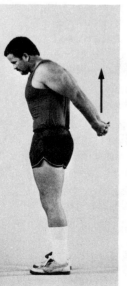

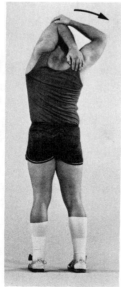

Hamstrings and low-
back stretch I

Hamstrings and low-
back stretch II

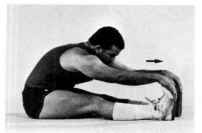

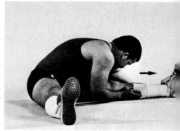

selecting a group of stretching exercises, you should include movements that work every joint from the feet and ankles to the neck and to the wrists and fingers. Of the vast number to choose from, pick stretching exercises that you like and that you won't skip because they're uncomfortable to perform. Some stretching may be done between exercises or at the end of a workout, as well as during warm-up.

Incidentally, I recommend that you do passive rather than dynamic or ballistic stretching. The passive method requires slow movement into the position needed to stress the joints and muscles being worked. Movement continues until you feel slight discomfort in the muscles or joint areas being stretched, at which point you hold the position for about 10 seconds. Relax slightly for 5 to 10 seconds, then start another period of stretching. Repeat this procedure several times for each joint or combination of joints being worked.

Ballistic stretching involves bouncing, with the momentum of other body parts forcing joint structures, such as ligaments and tendons, to elongate. The bouncing action also causes sudden stretches to be imposed on the associated muscles, with the possibility of a nervous system reaction called a "stretch reflex." This reflex facilitates contraction of the stretched muscle—just the opposite of the relaxation which is needed. In addition, "viscoelastic" proper-

Quadriceps stretch I

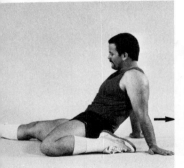

Quadriceps stretch II

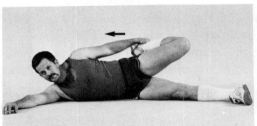

Spine and back muscles stretch

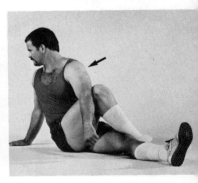

ties of connective tissue cause it to resist stretch more forcefully when pulled rapidly rather than slowly. Thus, ballistic stretching is physiologically untenable and may even result in tiny tears of the muscles and connective tissues involved.

A second type of warm-up, which can be just as important as general warm-up, is called specific warm-up. This is simply practicing the physical activity you are about to engage in, but at a low intensity. Sprinters run short distances from the starting blocks with less than maximal effort. Basketball players take shots and do lay-up drills before the game. Baseball players take batting practice. For strength training you begin any lifting exercise with relatively light weights before moving up to the heaviest load for that workout. General and specific warm-ups, including stretching, should totally prepare you physically for a productive period of exercise.

So much for warming up. The remaining properties of a quality strength and conditioning program are:

2. *The program is complete and simple.* This means that the exercises in your program should work all the major muscle groups in your body (completeness) and that as few exercises as possible should be used to accomplish this goal (simplicity). Completeness is desirable for balanced development, while simplicity is desirable to shorten the duration of workouts and permit higher intensity and better focus of available energy. Some advanced or specialized programs may violate this concept, but these are an exception.

3. *The components of the program are repeated periodically.* That is, the same exercises, or groups of exercises that work muscle groups in a similar way, should be done at regular time intervals. The classic three-day-per-week (Monday-Wednesday-Friday or Tuesday-Thursday-Saturday) strength program seems to work best for most beginners. The method of periodic repetition may become somewhat complex within the four- to six-day-per-week programs often used by more advanced trainees.

4. *The program is progressive.* This concept is usually misunderstood. It means, for strength exercises, that the weight you lift in a given exercise should be increased regularly but *not* continuously. One simple way to do this when on a three-day-per-week program is to have one heavy, one light, and one medium training day each week. The weights lifted on the heavy day are increased every few weeks, and this results in heavier weights on the light day and on the medium day, which are about 80 and 90 percent of the heavy day, respectively. Different methods of being progressive in a consistent way, while incorporating the technique of variability, are presented in Chapters 5 and 7. Some kind of variability must be incorporated into any type of training program

if progress is to be maintained. The same exercise done day after day and week after week will result in total adaptation of the body and a cessation of progress, or overtraining, and a decrease in performance. Knowledgeable runners, for example, run different distances at different paces (intensity) from day to day and week to week during a training cycle. During the cycle, however, the intensity tends to increase while the distance fluctuates less and less from the race distance being trained for.

5. *The program is compatible with the trainee's abilities and goals.* The severity of your program should match your physical and mental capacities. If the program is not stressful enough, little or no adaptation will occur; if too stressful, you may not recover from your workouts and you may become "overtrained." A frequent error is for a beginner to copy the program of an advanced athlete or bodybuilder from an article in a periodical. Likewise, the components of the training program should be designed to match the desired end result. A high jumper trains differently from a distance swimmer or someone who is training only to improve general fitness. Some of the exercises may be the same, and the general principles on which the program is based may be the same, but the details will vary considerably. These ideas are considered in the circuit training example below and in Chapters 5 and 7.

To review, five basic characteristics of a quality strength and conditioning program are warm-up, completeness and simplicity, periodicity, progressiveness, and compatibility. Reasons for unsatisfactory results from a training program can usually be related to a violation of one or more of these properties.

TWO BASIC SYSTEMS OF STRENGTH TRAINING: PRIORITY AND CIRCUIT SYSTEMS

The Priority System

Physical activity that produces and maintains an elevated heart rate of about 150 beats per minute for 20 minutes or longer will result in considerable cardiovascular (CV) conditioning for the average person. Typical weight training workouts are conducted in what is called a *priority system,* where one of several exercises included in the workout is completed (highest priority) before going on to the second exercise, and so on. Each bout of activity with a given exercise is called a set, and it consists of a number of repetitions (reps). In a priority system, three sets of 10 lifting reps per exercise is most common. During the activity period or set, the heart rate increases considerably, but it drops off rapidly during the rest between sets. The rest period is needed for partial recovery so that the weight can be lifted for the required reps in the next set. Experiment has shown that the heart rates of competitive weightlifters doing typical training lifts, which require simultaneous use of the large muscle groups in the leg, hip, back, and shoulder areas, fluctuate between 110 and 160 beats per minute, if rest intervals are kept at one minute. Fluctuations in this range for 15 to 30 minutes or more will produce CV benefits for most individuals, but not as extensive as would occur if the heart rate remained close to 150 for the same period of time. The reason most individuals obtain minimal CV benefit from priority system weight training is that they rest too long (three to five minutes or more) between sets, either so they can lift heavier weights or because they are lazy. There is a real need for such longer rest intervals when a heavy weight must be lifted for several reps in multiple sets to achieve the goals of a strength-oriented program.

The Circuit System

Most individuals, however, including even high-level athletes at certain times during a training cycle, want—indeed, need—more general conditioning for muscle endurance, strength, and cardiovascular fitness. If such is your case, you can use a procedure called *circuit training,* which you can modify in several ways to help you achieve specific goals.

A circuit for a workout consists of a collection of stations, each station being an area or piece of equipment for a chosen exercise to be performed. Not all stations need be for a weight lifting or a strength exercise—one could be for stretching or rope jumping. But the example that follows will consider only the former type of exercises.

The idea behind circuit training is that you go from station to station through the circuit and repeat the circuit a number of times. If the circuit is properly designed, so that the muscles principally used alternate somewhat from station to station, you can keep moving and maintain a high heart rate. There is no doubt that, for a given exercise in the circuit, you could lift more weight for a specified number of reps using the priority rather than circuit system. But, as pointed out above, the circuit method's purpose is to develop other components of fitness in addition to strength. Besides, the specificity of exercise principle tells us that you must sacrifice something in strength gains to achieve additional training benefits such as CV fitness and endurance.

As an example of the variety of goals that you can attain with circuit training, consider this circuit:

1. Leg press—for hip and knee extensors
2. Dumbbell rows—for lats, deltoids and elbow flexors
3. Leg curls—for hamstrings and calf
4. Bench press—for pecs, deltoids and elbow extensors
5. Situps—for abdominals and hip flexors
6. Hyperextensions—for spinal erectors

Instructions for performing the exercises in this circuit are given in Chapter 4. Note that it is a complete program since all major muscle groups are worked, and that it is simple since it involves only six exercises. This circuit can easily be done three days per week to satisfy the periodic repetition rule and can be made progressive in a number of ways that we'll discuss later. It would also be compatible with the needs of a variety of trainees at the beginning or intermediate level of experience in overload exercise.

You may now be wondering how many times you should go through a given circuit, how many reps you should perform at each station, how much weight you should use, and how much rest, if any, you should take between stations. The answers depend on whether you want to emphasize *cardiovascular fitness and muscle endurance* in your program or *strength development.* Making this decision is sometimes referred to as finding a training point on the strength-endurance continuum. To help you in your decision, and to tailor your program to your needs, you should understand that each type of program has its own characteristics. A CV and endurance-oriented program, for example, is characterized by:

1. Little or no rest between stations; or performing an activity like jogging in place, jumping jacks, jumping rope, or pedaling a stationary bicycle for 30 seconds to a minute between stations
2. Higher reps at each station (10–20)
3. Many excursions through the circuit (5–10)
4. Lower weights lifted at each station (relative to your maximum lifting ability)

By contrast, a strength-oriented circuit program is characterized by:

1. Rest periods between stations (about one minute)
2. Lower reps at each station (3–8)
3. Fewer excursions through the circuit (3–5)
4. Heavier weights lifted at each station (relative to your maximum lifting ability)

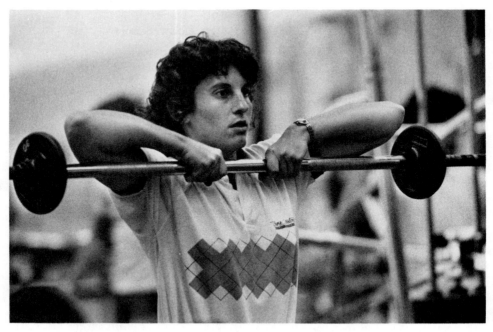

Circuit systems can be tailored to develop either cardiovascular fitness and endurance (more reps, less weight, less rest between exercises) or strength (fewer reps, more weight, more rest between exercises).

Some coaches who work with a large number of students or athletes at once will have one person start at each of the available stations and will signal when to start exercising, when to stop and rotate to the next station, when to start exercising again, and so on. This limits the number of reps at a given station by time and makes maximum use of available equipment. The weights used in this case should be adjusted by each of the individuals so that they can "keep going" during each exercise interval but are really working hard just before the interval ends. When a fixed number of reps is assigned at each station, the weight should be chosen so that the last couple of reps are difficult to complete, especially the final time or two through the circuit. This is especially true when the workout session is meant to be a heavy training day.

Circuit weight training is often called aerobic weight training. This is inaccurate. A muscle must be continuously active for more than about two minutes to shift primarily to aerobic metabolism, and since a circuit should be designed to alternate muscle groups from station to station, the time criterion is not satisfied. A significant amount of aerobic metabolism certainly occurs during the repetitive work-recovery cycles within a circuit program, but it is not generally the primary energy supply system while work (exercise) is being performed. The anaerobic (non-oxidative) energy system and stored ATP satisfy most of the muscles' energy needs during the work.

Note that weight machines are not needed to do circuit weight training. Indeed, though they make changing weight easy, they have some disadvantages as we'll see. In crowded public gyms and spas with limited equipment, you may find circuit training impractical due to use by other people of equipment you may need for one of your stations. If this is the case, you can orient a priority system toward an emphasis on cardiovascular fitness and endurance by doing higher rep sets with little rest between them, or by alternating just two or three exercises at a time rather than all exercises as in a single complete circuit.

Any circuit system that you set up should satisfy the five properties of a quality program given earlier. Training cycles (discussed in some detail in Chapters 5 and 7) can incorporate both circuit and priority training. You can, for example, train for a month or two on a circuit system with overall conditioning the emphasis, and then switch to a priority system for a similar period to build strength. The next chapter will discuss places to train and the advantages and disadvantages of various types of equipment. Chapter 4 will describe a large variety of strength training exercises that you can use to construct your program. Later chapters provide more detailed examples of programs and training cycles.

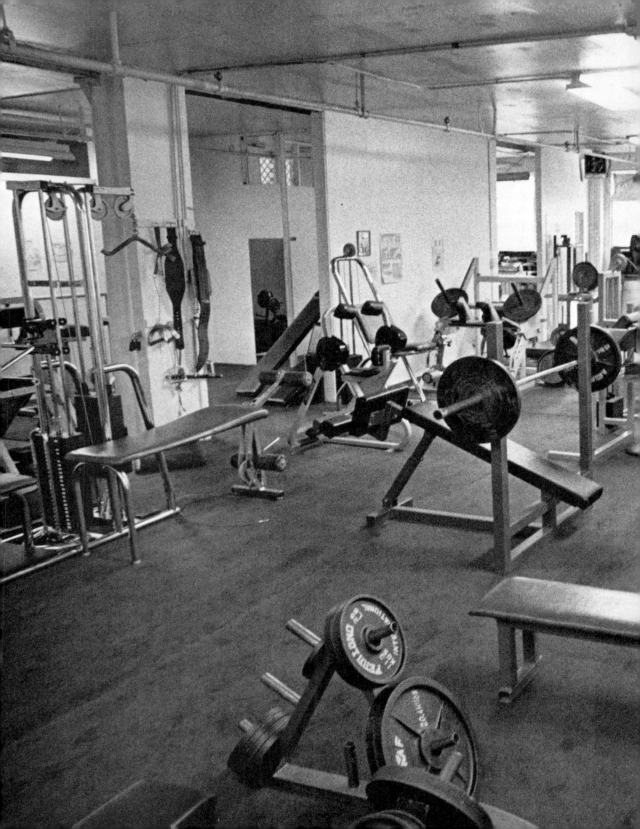

3

Strength Training Equipment and Places to Train

For decades, essentially the only strength training equipment on the market were "free weights"— barbells and dumbbells. Simple to use, durable, and relatively inexpensive, they fulfilled the training needs of "iron game" participants and strength fitness enthusiasts alike. Then, in the late 1960s and early 1970s, a variety of machines began to appear, with their manufacturers promising users more efficient exercise and faster strength gains. Today, companies such as Universal, Nautilus, Hydra-Gym, DynaCam, Marcy, and Paramount produce a variety of resistance machines for strengthening various muscles. The equipment designs and training principles promoted by each company vary widely, due to different interpretations of kinesiological principles, means of providing resistance, muscle groups to be exercised, production costs, and potential users. But there is no question that weight and resistance machines are here to stay.

FREE WEIGHTS VERSUS MACHINES

Both free weights and machines have distinct functional characteristics that can be

Well-equipped public gyms and spas contain both machines and free weights.

considered advantageous or disadvantageous depending on your physical condition, training goals, and training situation. Free weight use has many advantages relative to most common training circumstances. Free weight use requires you to balance both yourself and the weight, resulting in greater muscle utilization (prime movers, synergists, and stabilizers) and the development of better coordination during forceful exertions. This improves strength transfer to real-life movements, whether for recreational, sport, or work activities. By contrast, machines do almost all the balancing and stabilizing work for you. Free weights permit total freedom of movement for any given exercise, rather than the constrained and rigid movements that machines demand. You are thereby able to utilize your individual leverages to best advantage, just as you do in real-life movements. Free weights also permit you to perform a great variety of exercises rather than the few a given machine permits. This is very important because it means you can add variability to your conditioning program over a period of months or years.

Machines certainly provide substantial convenience and safety. You can usually adjust the resistance simply by changing the position of a metal pin. With common quick-lock collars, however, it takes only a few seconds to add or remove a weight plate from a barbell, and this changing of plates causes you to do bending and lifting movements that will contribute to your exercise program. As for safety, machines have some advantages over free weights. You can fall with a barbell, drop a dumbbell on yourself, or get stuck underneath a barbell when performing the bench press. These kinds of accidents should not happen if you use proper technique in your free weight exercises, handle reasonable weights, and use "spotters" during exercises such as the squat and bench press. But if you're not careful, these kinds of accidents can happen with free weights, while they're unlikely or impossible with machines. Of course, there is no guarantee you will *never* suffer an injury on a machine; people do smash fingers between the stacked weight plates and have been known to pull muscles just as easily while using machines as free weights.

To many, machines make the most sense for health spas and public gyms. With a sufficient number and variety of machines, a large number of people can go through a complete workout in a relatively short time, usually less than an hour. True, initial expense of furnishing a gym with a complete set of machines to service all the muscle groups of the body is very high. But with routine lubrication and maintenance, machines can function reliably for many years. Machines also have the advantage of staying in one place, while barbells, dumbbells, and weight plates tend to get scattered over available floor space. And the proper use of machines can be easily taught by a single knowledgeable instructor, which reduces a gym's supervision needs.

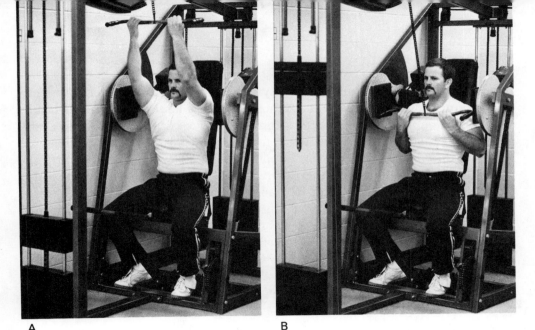

A   B

Most weight machines are designed to work specific muscle groups in isolation, or a few muscle groups together.

In short, machine training is convenient, safe, easy to learn, and productive in terms of exercise and increased strength. For many of you, these are the most important factors relative to your training goals and capabilities and available training time. But do understand that if you train only with machines, those compromises I mentioned a moment ago are always there: lack of development of balance and coordination during exertions, lack of variety in training movements over time, and constrained movement patterns. By being aware of them, you can take advantage of frequently overlooked methods to upgrade your overall training program—particularly by using a combination of free weights and machines in your program.

HOW MACHINES WORK

I think you'll find it interesting to know a little about how various resistance machines work and what's behind some of the claims their manufacturers make in sales advertisements. In using most of the common resistance machines you actually lift weights (part of a "weight stack") through some type of lever system. Any machine of this type can correctly be called a weight machine, with Nautilus and Universal machines being the most common examples. A lever system is a simple machine used to gain a positive or negative mechanical advantage. The most common lever system is the "first-class" lever, which can result in a positive mechanical advantage so that a large resistance *(R)* can be lifted with a relatively small effort force *(E)*. This occurs if the "lever arms" of *E* and *R* (the distances from each force to the pivot of the lever system) are adjusted to reasonable lengths. The actual lifting effect of your effort force *(E)* is equal to *E* multiplied by its lever arm length, as is the resistance *(R)* to lifting equal to *R* times its lever arm. This means that if your lever arm is five times longer than the resistance's, you can overcome a resistance up to five times greater than the maximum force you can exert. A first-class lever will always have a pivot or rotation point somewhere between *E* and *R*.

Levers

Example of a first-class lever system. Note that the pivot is in between the effort force (*E*) and the resistance (*R*).

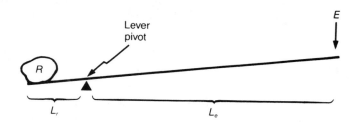

$$E \times L_e = R \times L_r$$

L_e = Lever arm of the effort force (*E*), which is equal to the distance from *E* to the pivot

L_r = Lever arm of the resistance (*R*), which is equal to the distance from *R* to the pivot

Example of a first-class lever system used in a leg press machine.

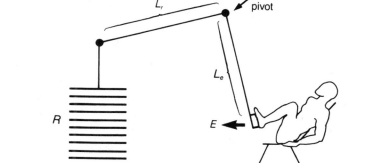

Example of a second-class lever system used in an overhead press machine. The pivot is at one end of the lever bar. The resistance (R) is a weight stack. If its attachment point (A) is designed as a rolling pivot, then the lever arm of the resistance (L_r) will change during the lifting movement —and the machine is then known as a variable resistance machine.

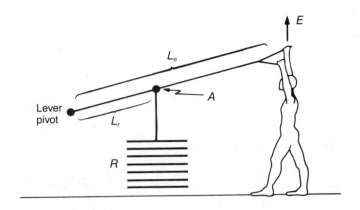

A "second-class" lever has a pivot at one end of a rigid bar. Effort is applied at the other end, and resistance lies in between. A wheelbarrow is the classic example of this type of lever system. The second-class lever always results in a positive mechanical advantage, since the lever arm of your effort force is longer than that of the resistance. Weight machine manufacturers most often use first- and second-class lever systems in their products.

Your body is composed primarily of "third-class" lever systems, which have an effort force (that is, muscle pull) in between pivot and resistance. The example shown below emphasizes the importance of muscle attachment variations. Consider only the biceps working to flex the elbow joint as illustrated. The example shows that, for a mere half-inch change in location of the bicep insertion point, a 33 percent increase occurs in the weight (R) that can be held in the hand for a given muscle tension. Hard to believe? The numbers don't lie. Because of the structure of a third-class lever (with E between R and the pivot, the lever arm of R is greater than that for E), the effort force exerted must be greater than the resistance lifted (negative mechanical advantage). The positive factor in this type of system is that the hand, for example, moves a considerable distance with even a short contraction of the bicep muscle.

Example of a third-class lever system in the body. Note that the effort (E) lies in between the pivot and the resistance (R).

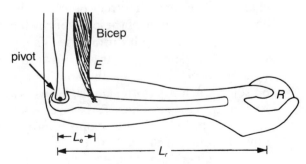

NOTE: If L_e = 1.5", L_r = 12", and E = 60 lbs. (muscle tension), then from $R \times L_r = E \times L_e$, $R = E \times (L_e/L_r)$ or $R = 60 \times 1.5/12$ = 7.5 lbs. If, instead, L_e = 2", then $R = 60 \times 2/12$ = 10 lbs.

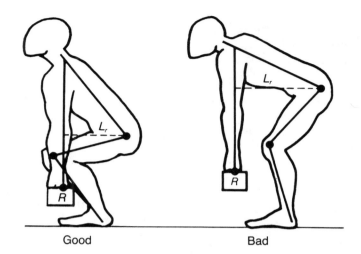

Lifting with the legs (good) rather than with the back (bad). The shorter the lever arm of the resistance (L_r), the less effort required of the lower back muscles.

Good   Bad

When you lift a barbell or other object from the floor, you should use your legs and not your back. Reason: When lifting with your back, you allow the object *(R)* a long lever arm. This results in your having to apply a very large muscle force in your lower back due to the short lever arm for the muscle effort, and can lead to injury and pain in your lower back area. As we'll see in the next chapter, this is the reason for emphasizing correct form in exercises like squats and pulls.

As movement occurs at any given joint of your body, the lever arm and direction of the working muscles' pull change, since the muscle attachment point moves relative to the joint pivot. Thus, not only does the ability of a muscle to generate tension change during movement due to length-tension and force-velocity properties, as mentioned earlier, but the effectiveness of muscle tension in producing movement varies as joint rotation occurs due to leverage changes. The manufacturers of "variable resistance" weight machines try to compensate for some of these factors by having the machines' lever arms change their functional length during use. This is typically done using a cam, which varies the distances from its axle pivot to the point where force is being applied by a chain or cable (as with Nautilus machines). A rolling pivot is also used on some machines (for example, Universal) to alter the ratio of the effort force lever arm to the resistance force lever arm during movement. But these variable resistance techniques at best only approximate changes in the ability of various muscle groups of the body to produce force. The five-foot, 100-pound gymnast certainly differs as a strength trainee from the seven-foot, 250-pound basketball

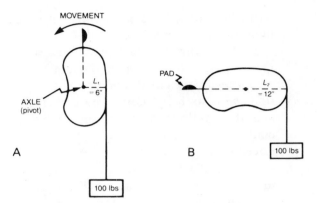

Cam method for varying the force required to lift a fixed weight.

At position A the turning effect caused by the 100 pound weight is 600 inch-pounds (100 x L_1 = 100 x 6). As the cam is turned by pushing on the pad the lever arm of the weight increases. At position B the turning effect is 1200 inch-pounds (100 x L_2 = 100 x 12). Since the lever arm from the pad (where you push) to the axle is a constant length as the cam turns, you must apply a greater and greater force to keep it moving.

player in limb and torso lengths and other variables, including muscle attachment points. All of these variables are important in the design of a training device. Machines are designed to average specifications and *cannot* be expected to match everyone's body characteristics exactly. You should consider these limitations when reading or listening to the advertising claims of machine salesmen.

Machines and Speed of Movement

Speed of movement, and its importance relative to training and the force-velocity relationship, is generally ignored by machine manufacturers. Nautilus recommends that all exercises be done slowly to keep this factor constant. As you will see in Chapter 5, however, the specificity-of-exercise principle indicates that *strength training with only slow movements and minimal accelerations does not transfer well to real-life activities,* especially in sport and recreation where fast movements are the rule.

"Isokinetic" Machines

We have talked about *concentric, eccentric,* and *isometric* contractions (Chapter 1). Some newer resistance machines, such as those produced by the Cybex and Mini-Gym companies, claim to permit an "isokinetic" contraction. The term "isokinetic" indicates constant speed of motion. Different frictional or hydraulic mechanisms are used by different companies to keep the movement speed fixed during various exercises. Some machines permit a range of movement speed settings from zero (isometric) to very slow to fast. Many isokinetic machines are well made and useful in controlled strength testing and rehabilitation owing to their ability to measure force through a full range of joint motion and at several speeds of movement. Some, however, are poorly made, do not control movement speed accurately, and can at best be classified as training novelties or gimmicks. If a given machine functions well at higher movement speeds, it can be helpful in teaching individuals how to make an explosive muscle contraction. Still, despite isokinetics' usefulness for specialized purposes, its value in general training is limited. Exercising at constant movement speed means, by definition, that no acceleration is present. All sport, recreational, and work activities involve considerable accelerations or changes in movement velocity. Thus, isokinetic exercise is not specific to real-life movement patterns.

Recent research studies have also shown that even the better designed isokinetic machines, when set to operate at higher velocities, maintain constant movement speed over only a small portion of the total range of movement. Part of the reason is that these machines don't begin to offer any resistance until the pre-set movement speed is reached, which, at higher velocity settings, may not

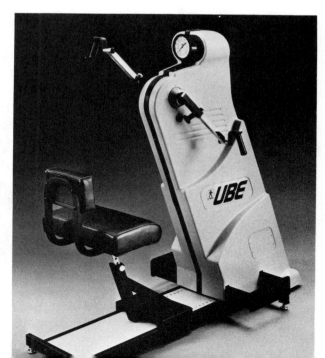

Isokinetic machines are designed to maintain a fixed movement speed during exercises. Some include a range of movement speed settings.

occur until a person is halfway through the movement range. So, although these machines are said to provide "accommodating" resistance, in that they are supposed to adapt to applied forces such that they move at a constant speed, they do so only during a part of the exercise movement.

Free Weights and Speed of Movement

Such problems do not exist when lifting free weights. Barbells and dumbbells always offer *at least* a resistance equal to their weight. Further, as you exert more and more force on a free weight, it will accommodate your effort according to the well-known engineering principle called Newton's Second Law of Motion. Simply, *the total force you exert on the bar will equal the weight itself plus a variable acceleration factor.* Thus, the free weights accommodate your lifting effort by accelerating at different rates, as occurs in real-life movement. And remember, everyone's lifting effort or force output changes during an exercise movement due to leverage changes and other factors. In stronger leverage positions you can exert more force and the bar moves faster (accelerates); in weaker leverage positions you can exert less force and it slows down (decelerates).

In some exercises you must voluntarily decrease your force output so that the barbell or dumbbell will slow down as you reach the end of the movement range. This occurs, for example, in elbow curls and dumbbell flys (described in the next chapter). In exercises of this type, where joints or dumbbells are coming together, variable resistance machines may offer an advantage since you can exert closer to a maximum force through a greater portion of the movement range due to the increasing resistance of the machine, which helps to slow the movement down.

Lifting free weights is often referred to as "isotonic" (constant tension) exercise. This is totally inaccurate, since while you lift a free weight the tension in any muscle being exercised is constantly changing. *Dynamic* exercise is a much more appropriate term for training with free weights, since it implies both movement and acceleration.

WHERE TO TRAIN: THE HOME GYM

Many individuals, including world-class athletes, do their strength training in a home gym. Before you decide to pay a substantial membership fee at the local health spa, look around you: Your garage, basement, or extra room may have great potential as a gym. Advantages are numerous and include: enjoying freedom from the hours and crowds of a public gym—you can train when you want; saving time by eliminating travel; always having the proper gym clothes readily available; getting family or friends involved as training partners; being able to do other household tasks, such as the laundry, while working out.

What You'll Need

If you find the home gym concept agreeable, you'll have to acquire certain basic equipment. You probably won't want to spend the money and don't have the space for the machines found in most public gyms. But don't worry. If you can equip your home gym with a barbell, dumbbells, and a variety of weight plates, you'll have essentially all the weight equipment you'll need to build your muscles efficiently. When buying weight plates, keep in mind that metal plates, though more expensive than the plastic-covered variety, last longer. Your choice should depend on how hard you'll use the equipment and how much weight you expect to need on the bar for your heaviest exercises. Plastic-coated weights are thick, making it difficult or impossible to get more than about 150 to 200 pounds on a typical exercise bar. With regard to bars themselves, check on the strength or maximum load capacity of any you consider buying. Some exercise bars are not solid steel and may be able to hold only 150 to 200 pounds before bending. This type of information should be available at the place where you buy the equipment.

If you are a stronger or more serious home trainee, you might consider spending more for an Olympic-style barbell set. Its bar is about seven feet long, permitting extra room for adding plates, and its plates have holes slightly over two inches in diameter, rather than about 1⅛ inches as with standard exercise plates. Whatever type of weight set you buy, be sure the total weight adds up to enough for your heaviest exercises, and that you have a good mixture of plates (1¼, 2½, 5, 10, 25 pounds) so you can load your bar or dumbbells in 2½-pound increments. Many barbell sets today come in the kilogram (kilo) rather than pound system. One kilo equals about 2.2 pounds. An easy way to convert kilos to pounds is to double the kilo weight and add 10 percent of that total. For example, 40 kilos equals 40 times two, or 80, plus 10 percent of that, or 88 pounds in all.

Besides a barbell, dumbbells, and weight plates, your home gym should have a padded bench, preferably one that can be inclined as well as used flat, and an adjustable-height rack, or set of supports, from which to lift the barbell

Equipment for the Home Gym

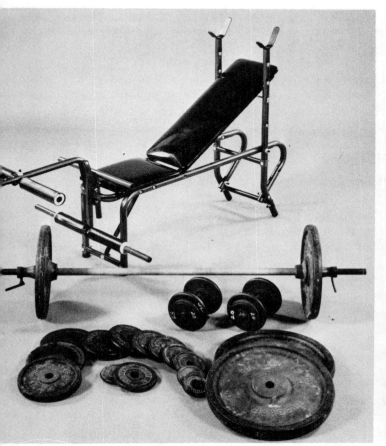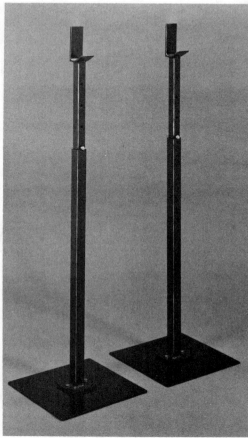

A barbell, dumbbells, weight plates, a padded bench, and an adjustable-height rack are all you need for a complete home gym.

Weight boots are an inexpensive alternative to a bench with a leg-extension, leg-curl device.

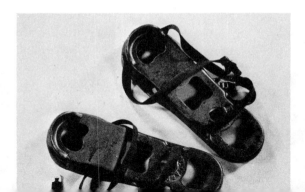

for certain exercises, such as the squat. If your bench doesn't have a leg extension-leg curl attachment, then a pair of adjustable weight boots will permit you to perform specialized leg exercises. A pulley device attached to the wall or ceiling is also useful for some specialized exercises, but certainly not required.

So this is all you really need to have a gym that will permit you to satisfy all the properties of a quality exercise program and allow you to make good progress. And its cost isn't outrageous: under $200. If you really want to economize, check the classified ads in your local newspaper for used equipment.

Machines for Home Use

If you're considering the home gym option, you've probably seen ads in magazines and elsewhere for resistance training devices that are, or resemble, health club–type machines but are promoted for home use. These devices fall into one of two categories: 1) actual *machines,* one example being Soloflex, and 2) *structures* (usually tubular steel) designed to permit a variety of exercises with barbell and dumbbell equipment, such as the Sears "home gym." The machines may use elastic cords, springs, air compression cylinders, or some form of weight plates to provide resistance. Before buying any home gym machine, you should consider how many exercises are possible for the numerous muscles of your body, and how well-built the machine is relative to its cost. The variety of exercises shown in the next chapter will help you answer the first part of this question. You must then decide if a given machine will meet your needs, permit you to exercise all the major muscle groups of your body (with or without additional equipment), permit variety in the exercises over time, and hold up under the wear and tear you'll give it.

The second category of home gym devices, like the Sears "home gym," usually allow for a greater variety of exercises than the first category, since they involve the use of barbells and dumbbells. Pulley systems that use the same weight plates are generally included on the device structure. Still, there are important questions you should ask before purchasing one of these devices. First, does the size of the structure and its components match your body size and limb lengths so that you can exercise comfortably? Second, do the pulley systems work smoothly with the amount of weight you would use? Third, is the structure built to last under the use you'll give it? Your needs and goals will dictate whether either category of home gym device is for you, or if a barbell, dumbbells, a bench, and a squat rack are all you need.

Home gyms, though great for some, cannot satisfy everyone's needs and desires. For example, you may not have the space at home to establish the type of workout area you want. If this is the case, you should probably consider joining an exercise club of some kind. The cost of a first-time, one-year membership at a typical health club or YMCA is generally comparable to the cost of basic home gym equipment. Many of you will enjoy the social aspect of training with others at a public gym. Maybe there is a gym close to your home or school or workplace that would make training stops convenient. Perhaps you enjoy training with certain equipment that is available at public clubs but too expensive for a home gym.

If you decide to join a public gym, you should consider two very important factors besides cost and location.

First, *determine the extent and quality of instruction available.* You can do this by talking to one or two of the instructors (not the membership salesperson) who work the hours you plan to train. Ask questions relevant to your needs and training goals. Consider whether the answers seem reasonable compared to what you know from your own reading and experience, or from what other qualified people have told you. Be wary of instructors who hesitate to talk to you or who "beat around the bush" rather than respond directly to your questions. But remember to be considerate of the demands you make on their time—they do have club members who need and are paying for supervision. Also, talk to others training at the gym to determine their feelings about and experiences with available instruction and supervision. A frequent complaint of people using public gyms is the lack of available and knowledgeable instructors. Let's hope this book makes you largely independent and able to develop your own training program. But public gyms generally have specialized equipment that requires instruction for proper use, and sometimes you'll find one or more exercises that you have difficulty learning to perform correctly. Or there may be instances when you unknowingly do an exercise incorrectly. These are all times when the presence and availability of a knowledgeable instructor is of considerable value. This consideration is also important if you plan to use a home gym. If you are even slightly unsure about how to perform a given exercise correctly, seek outside help from a knowledgeable acquaintance, or pay for instruction through a public gym or by private arrangement with a professional fitness instructor or strength coach.

Second, *look very closely at the type, quantity, and variety of equipment*

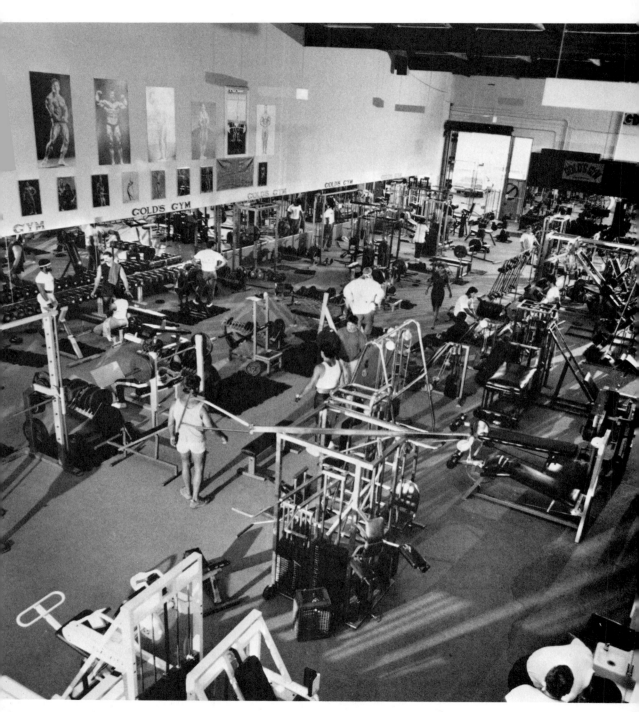

Gold's Gym, Venice, California, offers the best in both free weights and machines.

available at the gym you plan to join. If it has only one line of machines, such as Nautilus or Universal, that is a disadvantage. As the months go by, you will have almost no way of varying your training program. Variation is extremely important in producing continued adaptations to exercise, which means improvement. A given company's complete set of machines may permit only one or two basic exercises for a given muscle group. One or two exercises will not permit much variety over a period of months and years. If the gym you plan to join has some dumbbells and barbells available, in addition to a particular line of machines, the opportunity to vary your exercises as you progress is dramatically increased. The variety of exercises that can be done with barbells and dumbbells is almost limitless. A public gym with both machines and free weights offers the best of both worlds since you can mix exercises between the different types of equipment and alter this mixture periodically as the months go by. One only has to look at the bodybuilding mecca in Venice, California, known as Gold's Gym to see the incredible variety of machines and free weight equipment that the best public gyms can offer their members.

FINAL THOUGHTS

As you have probably guessed, the debate over free weights versus machines for strength training could go on and on. The considerations discussed above should help you make decisions about the equipment you will train on, whether at home or in a public gym. If you'd like more information on this question, Bill Starr, in his very informative text *The Strongest Shall Survive . . . Strength Training for Football,* devotes the eighteenth chapter to comparing free weights and machines relative to a variety of pertinent considerations. I should mention that his conclusions are very favorable to free weights, particularly as they apply to the training of athletes. In addition to Starr's text, there are several articles on this subject listed at the back of this book.

Finally, let's not forget the many strengthening exercises that can be done with essentially no equipment at all. Sit-ups and other calisthenics, such as push-ups and pull-ups, can all be used very effectively in many programs. A towel and a training partner can produce excellent conditioning exercises for the hamstring and neck muscles. Squeezing an old tennis ball regularly will strengthen the forearm muscles and grip. These and other often overlooked exercises are covered in the next chapter.

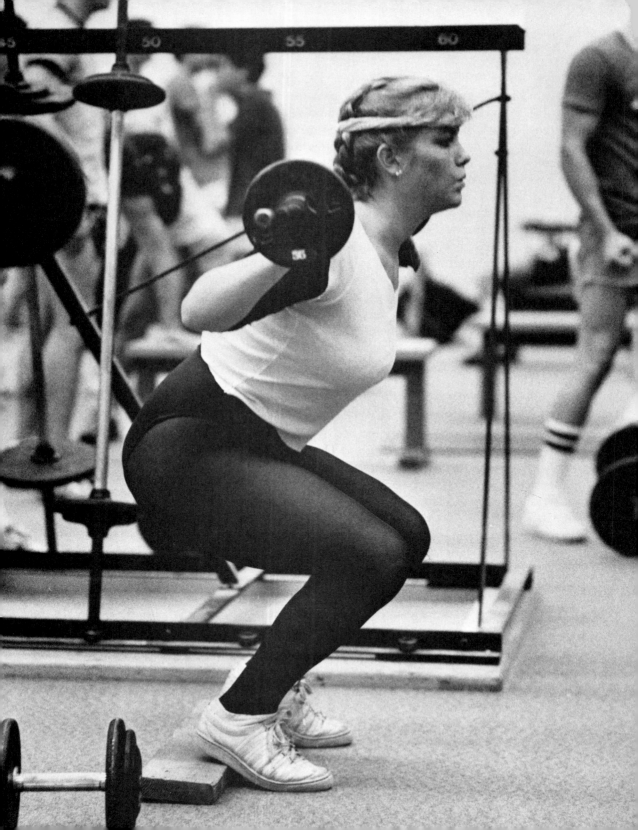

4

The Exercises

The components of any strength and conditioning program are its individual exercises. This chapter introduces many of the basic strength exercises that, through practical experience and kinesiological evaluation, have proven effective in building strength. The exercises composing your program could consist of countless combinations of those presented below. When you actually choose which exercises to do, however, never forget the need for completeness and simplicity, as discussed in Chapter 2. Also, it is extremely important that you learn to perform each exercise properly and that you are aware of which muscle groups are prime movers in the exercise and which others play a secondary role.

The exercises discussed and illustrated below are grouped according to multi-joint body regions that are involved in common movement activities, such as walking, running, jumping, or pushing. I call exercises involving multiple joints and muscle groups "core," or primary, exercises, since they are of primary importance and should form the major part of your program. Additional exercises that tend to isolate joints and muscles should be considered remedial, rehabilitative, or assistance-oriented and should play a minor, though often

63

Using proper breathing techniques is a must when strength training.

meaningful, role in your overall program. In some cases it is acceptable practice, based on the specificity of exercise principle, to modify the movement pattern of a given exercise so that it simulates the activity you are training for more closely. Be prudent, though. Trying an unsafe movement pattern can result in injury, and remember that the specificity principle does not imply that every strength training exercise must have exactly the same movement pattern as the activity you are trying to improve. As you read through the exercise descriptions below, be sure to study the illustrations. Learning to do the exercises properly is of paramount importance, and the combination of written descriptions and illustrations will help you understand precisely how to perform the movements.

An important point about breathing during essentially all strength training exercises: *Inhale just before* you start the exertion phase of the movement, *hold your breath during the exertion,* and *exhale at or just before completion* of the movement. Never hold your breath between repetitions of an exercise. By holding your breath during exertions, you "fix" your rib cage (that is, you hold it in one position so it is neither expanding or contracting). The rib cage acts as a foundation on which many muscles pull, and you don't want your foundation moving while your muscles are working vigorously.

Leg (Knee) Extension

Leg knee extension with a Nautilus machine
Start.   Finish.

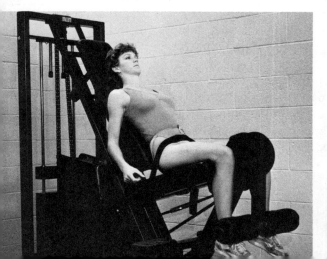 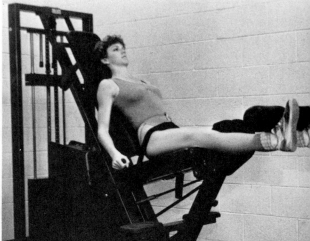

LEG AND HIP EXERCISES

Leg (Knee) Extension

Active Joint: Knee

Prime Mover: Quadriceps

Equipment: Leg extension machine, weight "boot" (preferably adjustable), or manual resistance

Proper Execution: From a seated position (using a leg extension machine) with your knees just over the edge of the bench, your feet behind the padded crossbar, and your hands holding onto the sides of the bench, slowly straighten (extend) your legs at the knee. Once you've reached full extension, slowly bend (flex) your knees to return to the starting position. During the lifting motion to full extension, the quadriceps perform a shortening (concentric) contraction, while during return to the starting position (when the weights are slowly lowered) the quads perform a lengthening (eccentric) contraction. Most of the exercises you perform with weights contain both a concentric and eccentric phase of muscle contraction. This is good news since it means your muscles have to work in two different ways during the complete exercise movement, resulting in the greatest training effect.

Knee extension with a weighted boot
Note that a higher bench or table will permit greater range of motion since the weights will not touch the floor.

A   B

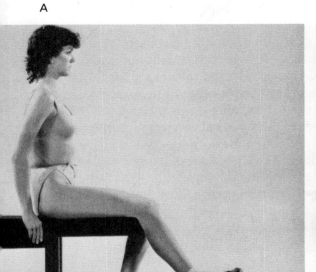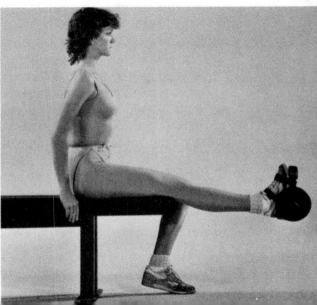

Performing this exercise with a weighted "boot" attached to your foot is essentially the same as with a machine. You simply sit on a bench or table and do the knee extension-flexion movement.

Likewise, when a partner manually provides resistance, he or she will kneel in front or to the side of the leg you are about to exercise while you sit on a bench or table. Your partner tries to push your leg into a more flexed position both while you straighten and rebend your knee, adjusting the force to permit a slow but steady movement up and back. In a sense, your partner accommodates your quad strength by how hard he or she pushes on your leg.

The advantage of knee extensions is that they are easy to do. The limitations are that they work only the knee joint and, since the resistance is applied near the ankle (a long lever arm distance from the knee), they produce large shearing forces that tend to make the bones at the knee joint slide away from each other. This is not a problem with reasonable training weights and their normal progression. Most other quad exercises, like squats and leg presses, produce less objectionable compression forces at the knee which press the bones together.

Leg (Knee) Curl

Active Joint: Knee

Prime Movers: Hamstrings

Equipment: Leg curl machine, weighted "boot" (preferably adjustable), or manual resistance

Proper Execution: Leg curls are the opposite of leg extensions. You can usually do them on the same machine, but this time, instead of sitting, you lie on your stomach. Some companies, such as Nautilus, have a separate machine for the leg curl. From the starting position, with your legs straight and ankles under the padded crossbar, slowly bend your knees until they reach the fully flexed position. Be sure your kneecaps are just over the edge of the bench when you start, so that the support pressure is felt on your lower quads above the knee joint. You don't want this pressure to push your kneecap against the bones of the moving joint, since the resulting friction may cause pain and injury. From the fully flexed position, slowly lower the weights by extending your knee until your legs are once again straight. As with the knee extension, your active muscles, this time the hamstrings, have gone through a concentric-eccentric (shortening-lengthening) contraction cycle.

You can perform the leg curl exercise with a weighted boot or boots while

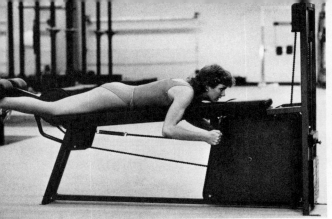
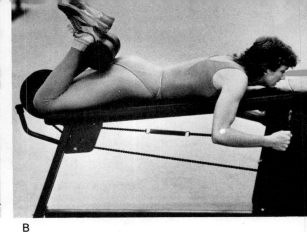

A   B

Leg curl (knee flexion) with a Nautilus machine
Start (A), finish (B) with maximal knee flexion. Note that the kneecaps should be just
over the edge of the bench.

lying on a bench or table with the kneecaps just over the edge, with or without
some padding (such as a folded towel or piece of foam rubber) under the lower
thighs. But I recommend doing them while standing (as shown in the illustrations), which is safer. Balanced on one leg, simply flex the other knee slowly
to bring the boot up as close to the buttocks as possible, then slowly return to
the starting position. If you do leg curls with a weighted boot(s) while lying on
a bench or table, be *very* careful to do the extension (leg straightening) phase
slowly so that you don't hyperextend your knee.

Leg curl with a weighted boot
Starting position (A), nearing the finish position or maximal knee flexion (B). The
range of motion can be extended by standing on some books or a block of wood
so that the weighted foot does not touch the ground at the starting position.

A   B

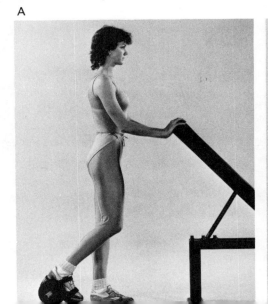
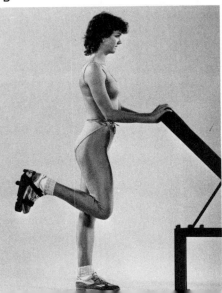

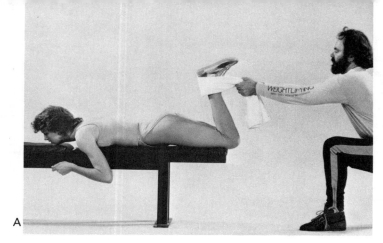

A

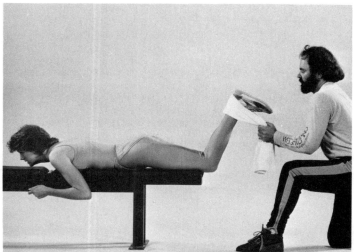

B

Manual resistance for strengthening the hamstring muscles
The trainee should resist knee extension (eccentric contraction)
as well as cause knee flexion.

Your training partner can also manually apply resistance as you lie face down on a bench or table by trying to pull your legs straight, with a rope or towel around your ankles, both while you flex and while you extend at the knee.

Leg curls are an excellent means of developing the hamstrings, and should always be included with exercises that develop the quads to maintain a level of balance in flexion-extension strength at the knee joint.

Calf Raise

Active Joint: Ankle

Prime Movers: Soleus, gastrocnemius

Equipment: Various machines, barbell, dumbbell, or manual resistance

Proper Execution: Any plantar flexion movement at the ankle joint that either raises the heel or lowers the ball of the foot can be considered a calf raise exercise. The exercise name comes from its most common form, namely, in a standing position, rising up on your toes by contracting your calf muscles. You can add extra weight by holding a barbell on your shoulders behind your head while you do the calf raises at a slow to medium speed.

To work different sections of the calf muscles, you can alternate sets, or even repetitions of the exercise, with the toes pointing first out to the side, then straight ahead, then inward. Another way to add resistance is to hold a dumbbell in your right hand when rising on the ball of the right foot and vice-versa. This frees your other hand to hold onto a bench or wall to help maintain balance.

Various types of "calf" machines found in gyms and spas also provide resistance during either a seated or standing calf raise motion.

Your training partner can even provide resistance by sitting on your lower back-hip area with you bent over at the waist, your legs straight, and your upper body supported by your arms on a bench or chair. This type of calf raise exercise is appropriately called the "donkey" calf raise.

To increase the range of motion at the ankle joint you can perform any of the above calf raise exercises with the balls of your feet supported on a board or weight plates one to two inches thick. You may not need to do calf raises if you do a lot of running or cycling in your overall conditioning program.

Five Calf Raise Exercises

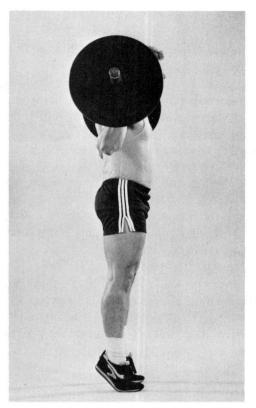

Calf raise with barbell on shoulders

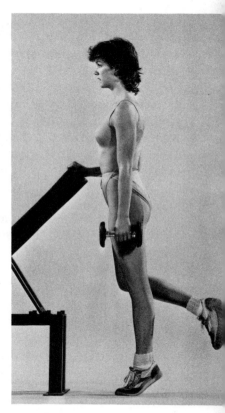

Calf raise with dumbbell held in ha

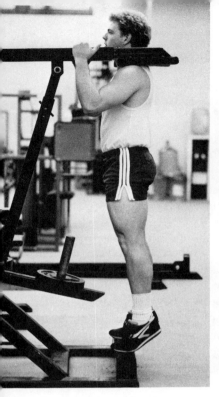

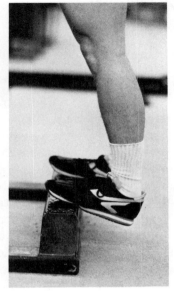

Starting position. You can increase your range of motion by standing on a board.

Typical calf-raise machine
Finish position.

Seated calf-raise machine
Note the third-class lever system (force applied between the pivot and resistance), as explained in Chapter 3.

"Donkey" calf-raises with a training partner providing resistance

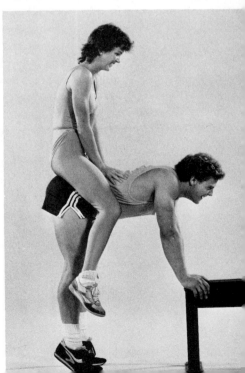

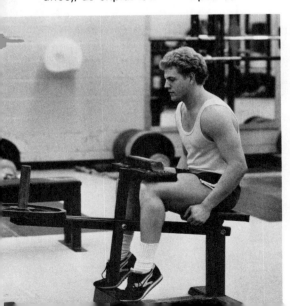

Hip Abduction-Adduction

Active Joint: Hip

Prime Movers: Gluteus medius and minimus, adductors

Equipment: Specialized machines, pulley devices, weighted "boot," or manual resistance

Proper Execution: Some companies sell specialized hip abduction-adduction machines, which provide adjustable resistance while you perform these hip movements from a seated position. If you don't have access to such a device, manual resistance is the simplest substitute.

While lying on one side on the floor or a bench, try to lift (abduct) your opposite leg as high as possible while your partner pushes downward between your ankle and knee. The force should be great enough so that you have to exert considerable effort to slowly lift your leg. Your partner should also push downward as you resist and slowly return your leg to the starting position. This results in your gluteus medius and minimus undergoing both a concentric and eccentric contraction.

The adductors can be strengthened by lying on your back on the floor or a bench, and repeatedly bringing your legs together (adducting) while your partner tries to push them apart. If you also resist your partner's push as your legs abduct to the starting position, you'll work your adductors eccentrically, in addition to the initial concentric phase.

You can use a weighted boot to exercise the gluteus medius and minimus by slowly abducting one leg at a time, either while standing or while lying on your side. Slowly return your leg to the starting position to work the abductor muscles eccentrically.

The adductor muscles are difficult to work effectively with weighted boots, so we won't consider such exercises. But pulley systems, in addition to manual resistance, can readily be used to exercise the adductor and abductor muscles. The cable from a pulley wheel located near floor level must be attached to your foot or ankle. Standing sideways to the pulley device, you can adduct or abduct at the hip, depending on which foot is attached to the cable, lifting the weights on the pulley system. The movement should be slow but steady.

Hip Abduction-Adduction

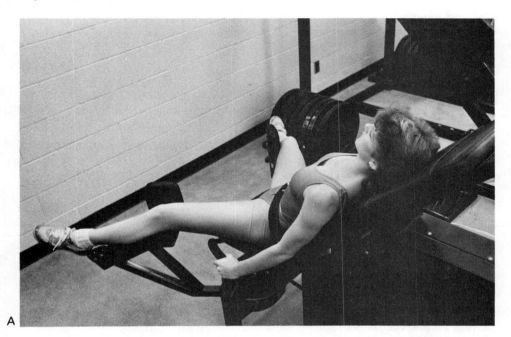

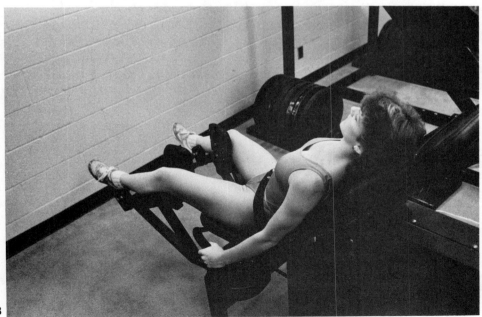

Hip abduction-adduction with a machine
This exercise can also be done with resistance supplied by a training partner, a pulley device, or a weighted boot.

Leg Press

Active Joints: Hip, knee, ankle

Prime Movers: Gluteus maximus, quadriceps, soleus, gastrocnemius

Equipment: Leg press machine

Proper Execution: There are actually several ways to perform the leg press exercise. Before the advent of weight machines, strength training enthusiasts would lie on the floor (usually with a pad or support under their hips) and have partners place a barbell on the soles of their feet, which they would then push upward (leg and hip extension) over their bodies for numerous reps. This method of doing the exercise certainly has obvious dangers, but nowadays I recommend the convenient (and safe) self-standing leg press machines.

In the past decade, the horizontally directed leg press machine—with a seat, foot pedals, and a weight stack—has become widely used. While seated and holding onto the sides of the "chair," you push the pedals forward with your feet until your legs are straight, thus lifting the attached weights via a lever system. This is an excellent exercise for all-around leg development since it involves the large extensor muscles at both the hip and knee, as well as the calf muscles. At the end of the push (as the knees straighten fully), the calf is activated when the balls of the feet are forced forward to plantar flex the ankle. The return to the starting position, with the hips and knees almost fully flexed, should be done slowly to work the gluteals and quads in a lengthening contraction. The seats on leg press machines are almost always adjustable so that you can position yourself at different distances from the foot pedals for the start of the exercise. The closer you are, the greater the range of hip and knee motion, but don't overdo it; you should feel comfortable in the starting position, not "squashed."

(NOTE: This is a good place to introduce you to a kinesiological concept we haven't yet considered. In multiple joint exercises, such as the leg press, muscles sometimes seem to work against each other. In the leg press, for example, the hamstrings aid the gluteus maximus in hip extension when you straighten your legs, while the quads extend the knee. But remember that the hamstrings also cross the knee joint from behind and tend to flex the knee when they contract. Thus, the quadriceps must overcome the hamstring's flexion tendency at the knee during the leg press. The quads are thus "dominant" in this particular movement situation. The resulting tension on both sides of the knee helps to stabilize the joint. Similar situations often occur at other joints of your body.)

The Leg Press with a Machine

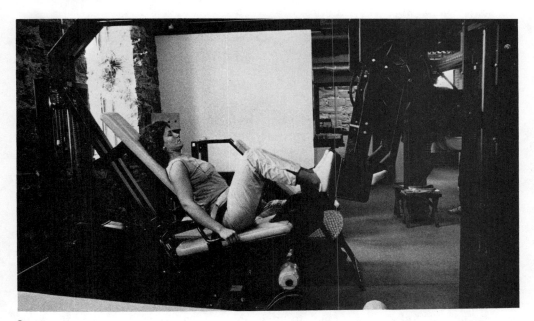

Start.

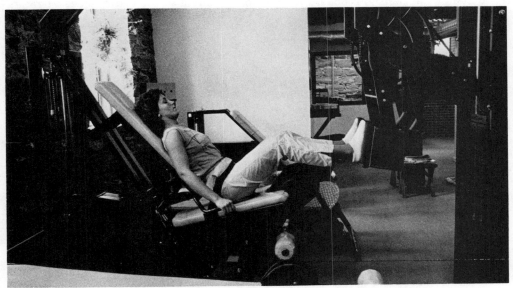

Finish.

Here, the trainee uses a horizontally directed leg press machine. Leg movement is smooth and slow.

Lunge

Active Joints: Hip, knee, ankle

Prime Movers: Gluteus maximus, quadriceps, soleus, gastrocnemius

Equipment: Barbell or dumbbells

Proper Execution: This exercise is usually done with a barbell held on the shoulders behind the head. Movement begins from the standing position, feet side by side, and the back is kept straight and tight throughout the exercise by isometric contraction of the spinal erectors. Start by taking a long stride forward with either foot, and then slowly lower your body as far as possible by bending the knee and hip of your stride leg (eccentric contractions of the prime movers). You can tell if your initial step forward is about the right length by noting if your lead knee is approximately over the toes of your lead foot at the

The Lunge

From the starting position (A), step forward (B). Your forward foot makes contact with the floor (C), and you slowly sink to the lowest position in the movement (D). Note that the front knee goes no farther forward than directly over the front toes. To return

A

B

C

D

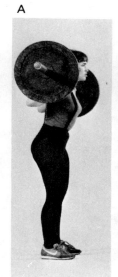
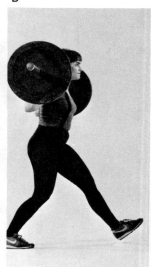
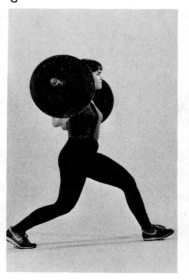
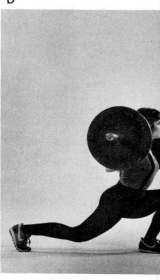

lowest position during the lunge. If it's back over your ankle, your step was too far forward or you haven't lowered yourself enough—maybe because your flexibility is poor or you didn't feel balanced as you lowered your body and you stopped too soon. Flexibility and balance can be developed with practice, so this first fault in knee position is common and can be easily corrected over time. If your lead knee is several inches or more in front of your toes at the lowest point of the lunge, however, you have not stepped forward far enough, and you must correct this error right away to avoid developing excessively large forces around the knee joint. Now, to complete the exercise, reverse the movement by pushing back off your lead foot (concentric contractions of the prime movers) and stepping back with two or three shorter strides until your feet are again side by side. I recommend alternating right and left foot strides, although some advanced trainees do 5 to 10 consecutive lunges with one leg before shifting to the other.

to the starting position, push up and back with the lead foot (E), then step back with the lead foot (F). Usually two smaller backward steps with the lead foot work best to bring you back to the starting position (G).

E

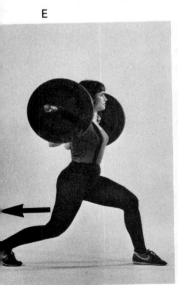

F

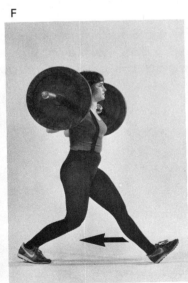

G

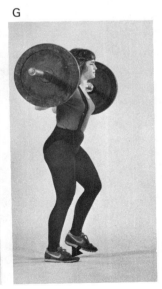

The dumbbell lunge
Start with feet together, hands holding dumbbells at sides (A). Step forward (B), and slowly sink to the lowest position in the movement (once again, the front knee has not moved any farther forward than over the front toes). From this position, step back as you would when completing a lunge with a barbell.

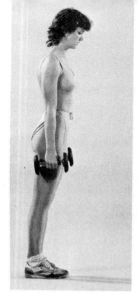

A

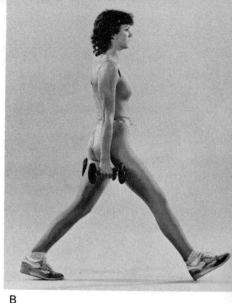

B

Though the same leg and hip muscles are used in the lunge as in the leg press, the lunge has an added benefit since it requires total body balance and coordination, resulting in the use of many torso and shoulder muscles not involved in the leg press. The idea of having to maintain body balance and coordinate total body movements while lifting weights is very important, since in normal daily activities (such as carrying a bag of groceries up stairs) and recreation, your body works as a whole, not in parts. This is why the lunge and other "total body exercises" discussed later in this chapter can be so valuable in your program.

If you are a beginner, you can learn the lunge more easily if you hold dumbbells in your hands rather than a barbell on your shoulders. This way, you minimize balance problems but still develop a feel for the demands of the

A

Stepping forward after lunging
From the lowest lunge position (D on pages 76–77) push forward with the rear foot, push up and pull back with the lead leg (A), bring the rear leg forward (B, C) and finish (D), ready to step forward with the opposite leg if space permits.

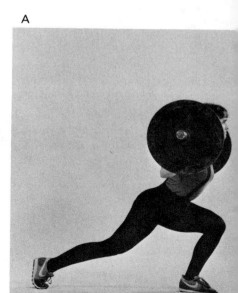

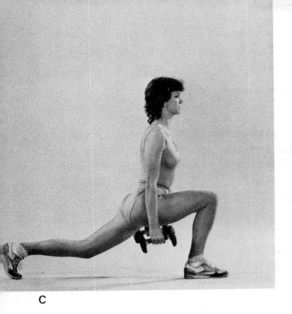

C

exercise (and develop grip strength at the same time). With either method, start with little or no weight and gradually increase the load.

Some variations of the basic lunge include (1) holding the barbell on your shoulders and clavicles (as described for the front squat exercise later in this chapter) rather than behind your neck and (2) stepping forward rather than back after the initial forward lunge. Runners particularly can benefit from performing this stepping technique. From the lowest position, simply push upward with your lead leg (rather than backward as with the standard lunge), while pushing forward with your back leg to complete the forward step. If you have enough space you can keep stepping forward and make several lunges, but if your space is confined, just walk slowly backward to your starting location after each forward lunge.

B   C   D

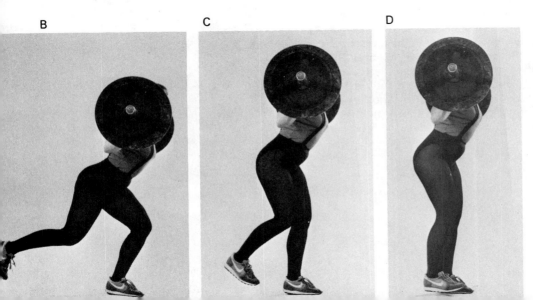

UPPER BODY "PUSHING" EXERCISES

The exercises listed below form an important group of movements, strengthening the arm, shoulder, and upper torso muscles used when pushing an object away from your body, or your body away from an object. Examples include pushing open a heavy office building door, pushing an opponent away in football or wrestling, and doing "push-ups."

Bench Press

Active Joints: Elbow, shoulder, shoulder girdle

Prime Movers: Triceps, anterior deltoid, pectoralis major

Equipment: Barbell or dumbbells, a flat bench; various machines

Proper Execution: The bench press is the most widely used strength training

The Bench Press

Start by holding the bar with hands wider than shoulders' width apart and at arm's length (A). Now slowly lower the bar to the chest near the base of the pectoralis major muscles (B).
Press the bar upward and slightly toward the head (C), until your arms are fully extended and the bar is in position for another repetition. Note the spotter in these pictures who can help the trainee in case of lifting problems.

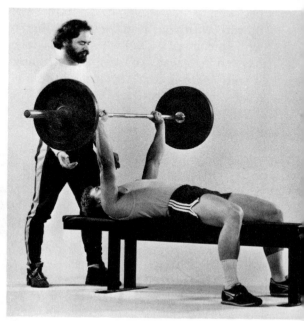

A

exercise in the United States and probably the world. This is largely because it's such an easy exercise to do and yet so quickly develops chest, shoulder, and arm muscles. You do the exercise while lying supine on a flat bench and using a barbell or one of many available bench press machines. Lying on the floor is not recommended since it does not allow you to lower your elbows past your torso and thus limits the range of your arms' motion and causes incorrect movement patterns. With a barbell, start the exercise by lying on a flat bench and either lifting the bar from the bench's supports, or by having a training partner hand the barbell to you so that you hold the bar above your chest with straight arms. Your grip should be a little wider than shoulders' width with your palms facing away from you. A good way to estimate proper grip width is to take the empty bar and bring it to your chest in the contact position as described below; if your grip is correct your forearms will be pretty much perpendicular to the floor rather than inclined out to the side or in toward your body. Small adjustments in your grip width are fine if they make the exercise movement feel more comfortable to you.

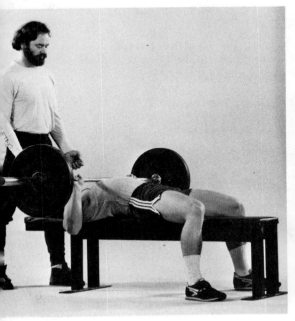

B

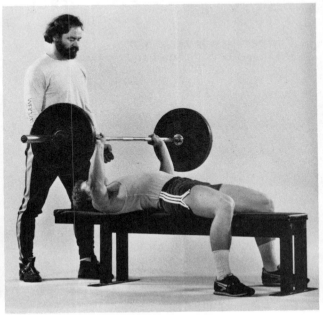

C

Bench-Press Variations

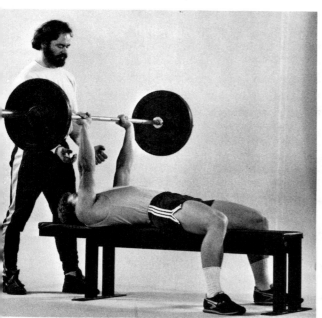

A

The narrow-grip bench press
(A) shows both the start and finish position.

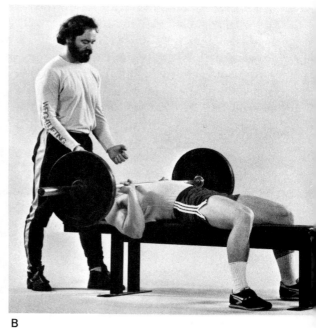

B

When the bar is at the chest (B), the elbows are kept in close to the body to simulate arm action in running.

The bench press with dumbbells
The dumbbells should be over the chest.

From the above starting position, with your upper back and buttocks firmly on the bench and your feet on the floor, *slowly* lower the barbell until it lightly touches your chest just above nipple level. Do not bring the barbell down rapidly and "bounce" it off your chest, and never bring it down to touch the upper chest near your neck. When the bar touches your chest, your elbows should not be in close beside your torso or pointing straight out to the side, but approximately midway between these two extremes. Some runners—particularly sprinters—keep their elbows in close to the torso during the bench press to simulate the proper arm movement pattern used in fast running. This is okay for such a special situation but is not recommended for beginners.

From the chest contact position, immediately push the barbell upward until your arms are again straight and holding the weight over your chest. The barbell should move upward from your chest in a *slight* curve toward your head rather than in a straight line. The upward lift should be slow to moderate in speed, although a faster upward movement speed can be used on lighter training days (as we'll see in Chapter 5). However, the *downward movement* should *always* be slow. Also, avoid lifting your hips off the bench ("bridging") while pushing the bar upward. This is a common method of "cheating" to lift more

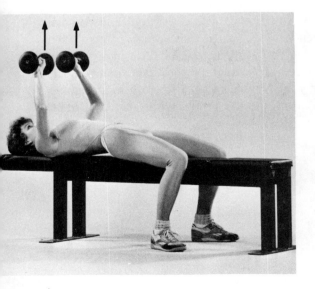

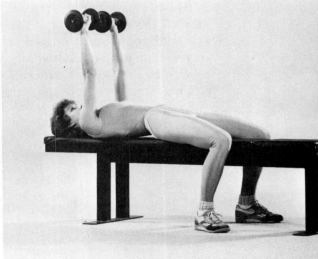

A   B

weight, but it prevents the proper working of the muscles for this exercise and can cause injury.

Finally, remember the proper breathing technique: Inhale either just before or as you start lowering the bar, and don't exhale until the end of the upward push for each repetition.

Lowering the barbell to your chest requires eccentric (lengthening) contractions from the prime movers, while the upward press requires concentric (shortening) contractions from the same muscles. If you use a narrower hand grip than recommended above, your triceps will be exercised more vigorously due to greater elbow flexion at the chest contact position. For some sports where triceps strength is especially important, this modified grip may be useful. The push-up exercise is similar to the bench press in terms of joint movements and muscles used, but the bench press allows you to change resistance more easily.

You can also hold a dumbbell in each hand and perform the bench press as described above. You'll find it a bit more difficult with dumbbells since each arm must control its load independently, making balance more of an effort than with a barbell. To begin the exercise, either lift the dumbbells to your shoulders, sit down on the bench, and slowly lie back, or lie down and have someone hand you one dumbbell at a time. During both barbell and dumbbell bench presses you should have a "spotter" stand behind you to help if you lose control of the weights or find yourself unable to lift the weights off your chest (known in weight training as "getting pinned"). This latter situation is particularly dangerous with a barbell, so a spotter is essential. Should you ever get pinned without a spotter, *don't panic.* Either tighten your abs and slowly roll the barbell toward your waist until you can sit up, or tilt the bar to one side and let it slide off your chest until one end of the bar touches the floor and you can slide off the opposite side of the bench.

With most bench press machines you perform the exercise in a position very similar to that used with a barbell. The machine, however, controls the balance and movement pattern for you. Nautilus and a few other companies produce bench press machines that allow you to exercise while seated upright.

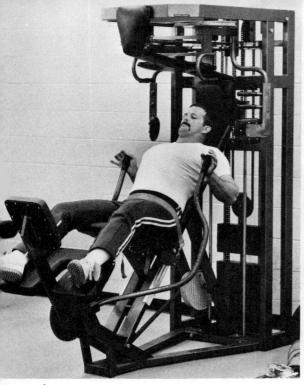

A

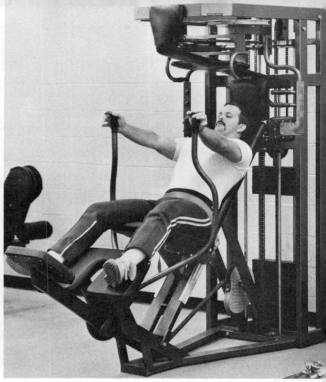

B

Bench press machines, such as the one shown here (A, B), and "pec" machines, such as (C), control the balance and movement pattern for you. Note the lack of elbow joint involvement with the "pec" machine.

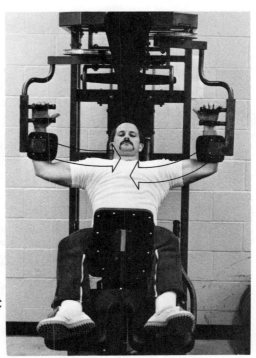

C

Incline Press

Active Joints: Elbow, shoulder, shoulder girdle

Prime Movers: Triceps, anterior deltoid, pectoralis major

Equipment: Barbell or dumbbells and an inclined bench

Proper Execution: The incline press is similar in most respects to the bench press described above, so this description will concentrate on the differences and not repeat the similarities.

The bench used is inclined up from the horizontal rather than flat. The amount of inclination is often adjustable from about 30 to 60 degrees. With most incline benches, you sit and lean back against the incline, although some are designed to allow you to lean back while you're standing.

If you're using a barbell, lift it from supports or a rack, or have it handed to you by spotters. In the starting position, hold the barbell over your upper chest with your arms straight and perpendicular to the floor, no matter what

A

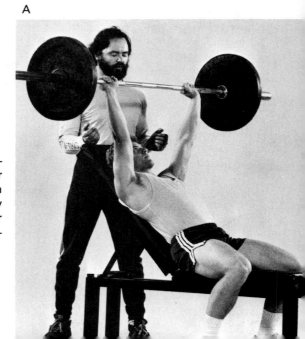

The incline bench press
(A) shows the start and finish position of the exercise. Slowly lower the bar to the upper chest (B), then press the bar upward and slightly toward the head (C). Use a spotter to assist you in case a problem develops.

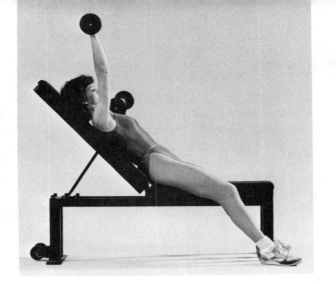

When performing the incline bench press with dumbbells, arms may be raised and lowered together, or alternately as shown here.

the bench incline angle. *Slowly* lower the bar to touch your upper chest or clavicles and shoulders. Then immediately push it back up to the starting position. Never let the bar "drift" toward the direction of your feet during the upward push or you might lose control of the bar and drop it. As with the bench press, spotters are very important when doing incline presses, but if you should get pinned without a spotter in the incline press, it is easier to sit up or stand and set the bar down than in the bench press.

B

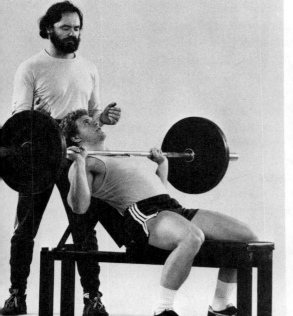

C

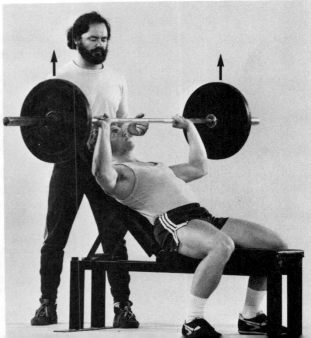

Muscle involvement during the concentric and eccentric phases of the incline press is similar to that in the bench press, except the upper portion of the pectoralis major is worked more extensively than in the bench press, where the lower portion of the pec is emphasized. The lower the incline of the bench (30 degrees, for example), the greater the similarity to the regular bench press. The higher the incline (60 to 70 degrees), the greater the similarity to the overhead press, which we'll discuss next.

As explained above for the bench press, dumbbells may be substituted for the barbell but it is generally difficult or impossible to replicate the incline press on a machine.

Overhead Press

Active Joints: Elbow, shoulder, shoulder girdle

Prime Movers: Triceps, anterior deltoid, trapezius

Equipment: Barbell or dumbbells; machines

Proper Execution: The overhead press requires pushing whatever resistance you're using upward from shoulder level to straight arms' length over your head. When using a barbell, begin either by lifting it from the floor to your shoulders (as described later in the "total body" pulling exercise section) or by taking it from a rack or set of supports on which you've placed the bar near shoulder height. Stand on the floor or sit on a bench or chair and hold the bar firmly across your shoulders and clavicles with your palms facing away from you. Keep your back and abdominal muscles tight (isometric contraction) as you push the bar upward at a slow or medium speed to arms' length overhead. You may have to tilt your head back at the start of the press so that the bar will not hit your chin, but never push the bar forward at the start of the press, only straight upward. Also, keep your spine straight to minimize any lean or backward bending (hyperextension of the spine) during the press.

Your triceps and anterior deltoids control elbow extension and shoulder abduction respectively (while your shoulder joints are externally rotated) via concentric contractions during the upward press. The trapezius muscle controls the upward rotational motion of your shoulder girdle as your arms rise overhead. Eccentric contraction of these same muscles permit you to return the barbell to the starting position in a slow, controlled manner.

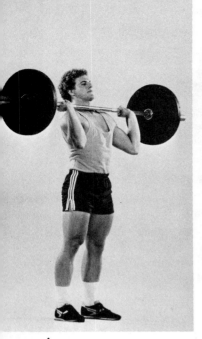
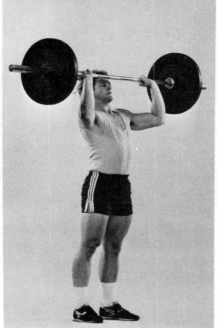
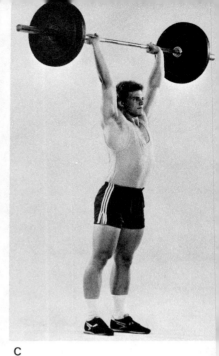

A   B   C

The standing overhead barbell press
Start with the bar at shoulder level (A), push the bar straight upward (B), finish with the bar directly overhead (C). Lower and repeat.

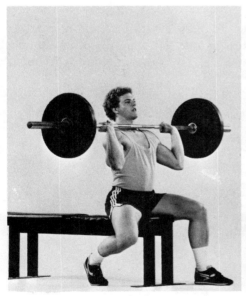
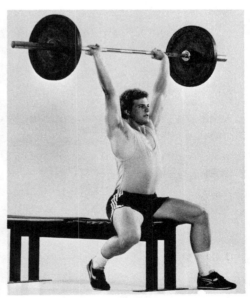

A   B

The seated overhead barbell press
Note how the trainee uses a split-foot position, which helps him maintain balance.

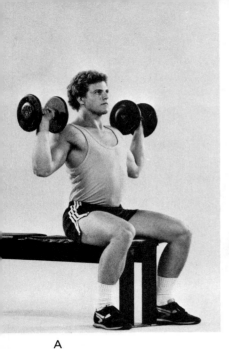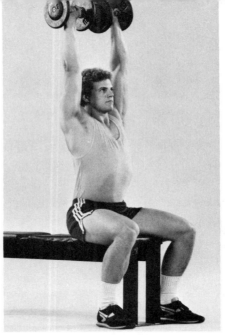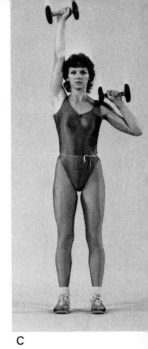

A B C

The overhead dumbbell press
You can perform the overhead dumbbell press either seated (A, B) or standing (C), with arms raised and lowered together (A, B) or alternately (C).

You can substitute dumbbells for the barbell with little or no change in the exercise technique, or alternate pressing one and then the other dumbbell overhead rather than both at the same time. This latter method is frequently preferred by beginners.

Several manufacturers produce machines for overhead presses. These are generally used in a seated position, and they control both your balance and your movement pattern.

Behind-the-Neck Press

Active Joints: Elbow, shoulder, shoulder girdle

Prime Movers: Triceps, anterior deltoid, trapezius

Equipment: Barbell or machine

Proper Execution: This exercise is similar to the overhead press, with the difference emphasized by the name "behind-the-neck press." Holding a bar in a starting position at the base of your neck, behind your head, press it slowly upward to arms' length overhead. Because of the starting position for this exercise, your shoulders are pulled back, which results in greater involvement of the trapezius in rotating your shoulder girdle upward as your arms rise overhead. Otherwise, though, the prime movers work concentrically and eccentrically just as they do in the regular overhead press. To get into the starting position, lift the barbell from the floor to your shoulders, as in the overhead press, and then slowly push it up and over your head and lower it behind your neck. Alternatively, you can simply lift it from supports or have training partners place it on your shoulders, as in the squat exercise (see "Total Body Exercises" later in this chapter).

Dumbbells are not effective for the behind-the-neck press movement since it is difficult to keep your shoulders pulled back due to the independent arm action.

Many overhead press machines can be used for the behind-the-neck press simply by facing away from the press bar when doing the movement rather than facing it as in the normal overhead press.

The behind-the-neck press
The bar starts and finishes behind the neck (A), and the bar is pressed to arm's length, slightly behind the head (B).

A   B

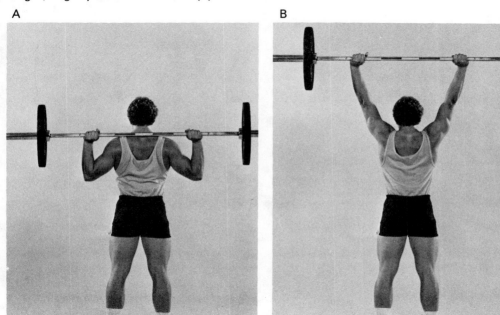

UPPER BODY "PULLING" EXERCISES

The exercises listed below form an important group of movements that strengthen the arm, shoulder, and upper torso muscles used to pull an object toward your body, or to pull your body toward an object. Examples include pulling open a heavy door, using your arms to help you climb a ladder, rowing a boat, doing a "pull-up" on a chinning bar, and many common swimming strokes.

Bent-Over Rowing

Active Joints: Elbow, shoulder, shoulder girdle

Prime Movers: Latissimus dorsi, posterior deltoid, elbow flexors

Equipment: Barbell, dumbbell, or pulley device

The bent-over row
The weight plates do not need to touch the ground at the start (A).

Raise the bar upward with your elbows moving slightly sideways (B).

Touch the bar to the lower chest (C) and return it slowly to the starting position.

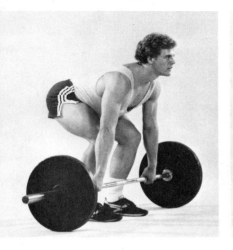
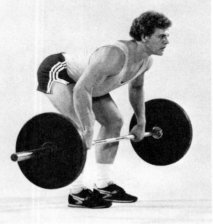
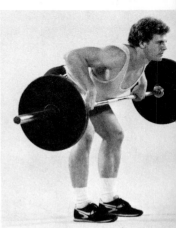

Proper Execution: With a barbell, use a grip a little wider than shoulder width —similar to what you use for the bench press described earlier. Hold the bar on your thighs with your palms facing you (pronated grip) while standing with bent knees. Lean forward, keeping your back straight and your head up, until your torso is about 30 degrees above the horizontal. With the bar hanging from your straight arms, pull it upward at medium speed until it touches your lower chest, then slowly lower it to the starting position.

With a dumbbell, the exercise position is similar, but one hand is placed on a bench or chair to help support the weight of your torso and reduce muscle tension in your lower back. Your other arm pulls the dumbbell upward from a hanging position until it touches the side of your chest just below the shoulder. Your elbow should be in and close to your body at this finish position, not out to the side. Slowly lower the dumbbell to the starting position. I recommend rowing with a dumbbell rather than a barbell for anyone with low back pain or back weakness.

Depending on the exact pulley system design you may have available to

The bent-over dumbbell row
Keep the elbow in and close to the body during the rowing motion, not out to the side.

A

B

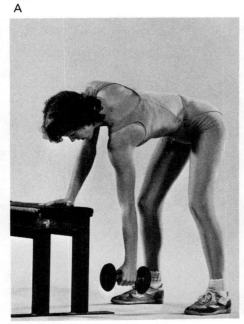
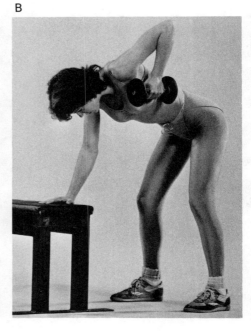

you, you can perform a rowing motion in a manner similar to either barbell or dumbbell rows, or seated on the ground, pulling the cable bar or handles horizontally toward your chest. Each of these methods requires a pulley system with a pivot wheel at floor level.

The prime movers in any rowing exercise contract concentrically (shorten) as you pull the resistance toward your chest, and eccentrically (lengthen) as you slowly lower the resistance. The "lats" (latissimus dorsi muscles) and posterior deltoids pull your upper arms backward from the starting position. Kinesiologists call this motion *transverse abduction* of the shoulder joint if your elbow moves out to the side, as with barbell rows, or *shoulder extension* and *hyperextension* if the elbow stays in close to your body, as with dumbbell rows. The biceps and other elbow flexors control motion at that joint.

Always do rowing exercises using the fullest possible range of motion. If

Horizontal rowing using a pulley device
As in the bent-over row, the elbows stay close to the sides during the rowing motion.

A

B

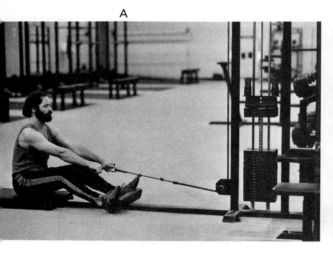
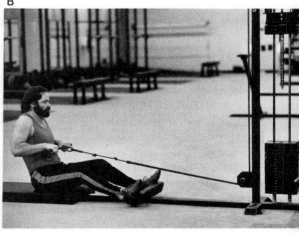

the weight is too heavy for you to pull it all the way to your chest, reduce it. Full range of motion causes the scapula to move extensively toward and away from your spinal column during the rows, and activates the rhomboid and lower part of the trapezius muscles of your upper back with shortening and lengthening contractions.

Some machines permit a "pulling-in" motion that falls between a true rowing motion and the "lat" pull-down motion we'll discuss below. You can make a simple rowing "machine" by loading only one end of a bar and wedging the other end into a corner. Stand over the loaded end of the bar, bend your knees and grasp the bar just behind the plates. Now, while looking forward and keeping your back tight and straight, "row" the weights at a moderate speed up to your chest and back to the starting position.

A simple rowing machine using a barbell

A

B

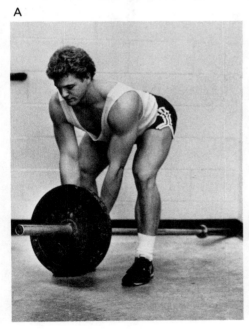 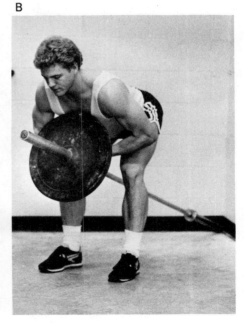

Upright Rowing

Active Joints: Elbow, shoulder, shoulder girdle

Prime Movers: Trapezius (upper parts), deltoid, elbow flexors

Equipment: Barbell, dumbbells, or pulley device

Proper Execution: Stand erect and, with arms straight, hold a barbell at your thighs, with your palms facing you (pronated grip) and about four inches between your index fingers. Pull the bar upward along your body at slow to moderate speed until it reaches your chin. As the bar moves upward, your elbows move up and out to the side (laterally). Slowly lower the bar along your body to the starting position until your arms are straight.

The middle and posterior parts of your deltoids control the shoulder movements (abduction and adduction while rotated inward or medially) via concentric contraction upward and eccentric contraction downward. Likewise, the upward and downward gliding action of your shoulder girdle is controlled by the upper parts of your trapezius muscle. The elbow flexors control motion at that joint.

You can do this exercise in an almost identical manner using dumbbells, or standing close in front of the floor-level pivot wheel of some pulley devices and rowing the cable bar or handles up along your body to chin level.

The Upright Row

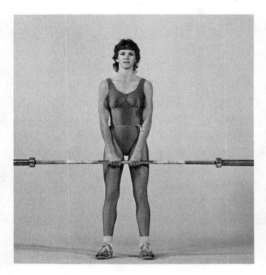

Starting position (A).

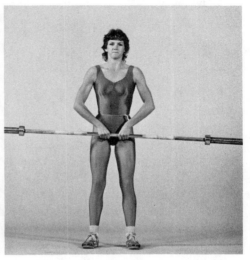

As you pull the barbell upward, your elbows should move laterally rather than backwards (B).

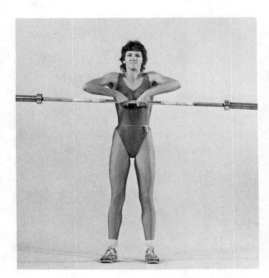

As you continue to raise the bar, keep it close to your body (C).

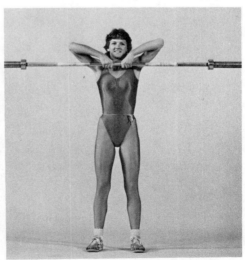

At the finish, the bar should almost touch the chin (D). Now slowly lower the barbell to the starting position.

Lat Pull-down

Active Joints: Elbow, shoulder, shoulder girdle

Prime Movers: Latissimus dorsi, pectoralis major and minor, rhomboids, elbow flexors

Equipment: Overhead pulley device

Proper Execution: Overhead pulley devices are usually called "lat" machines, since they are most commonly used to perform the lat pull-down exercise to develop the latissimus dorsi muscles. You should sit or kneel directly under the pulley and, using an overhand grip considerably wider than shoulder width, pull the bar from arms' length overhead down to shoulder level behind your head. Then, slowly let the weight pull the bar upward as you resist until you are again in the starting position.

This method works the prime movers during both shortening and lengthening contractions. The upper arms are pulled down (adduction of the shoul-

The behind-the-neck lat pull-down
The trainee is using a wide-grip bar with a pulley system.

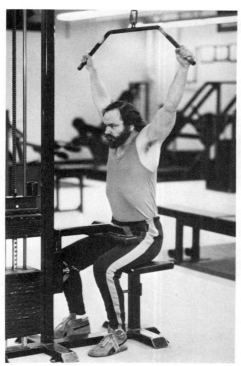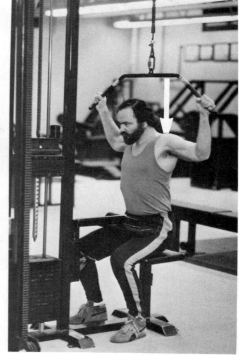

A   B

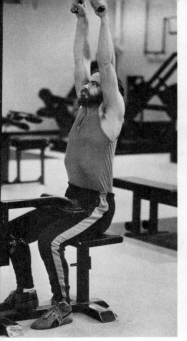 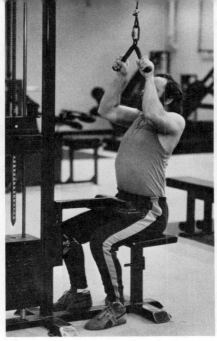 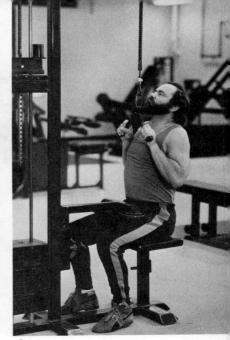

A   B   C

The lat pull-down to the chest
The trainee is using a narrow-grip bar with a pulley system.

ders while they are rotated externally) by concentric contraction of the pecs and lats. Likewise, the shoulder girdle rotates downward by contraction of the rhomboid and pectoralis minor muscles, while the elbow joint flexes due to contraction of its flexor muscles. If you pull the bar down to your upper chest rather than behind your head, the pectoralis major is worked harder. Relative to muscle and joint action, these pull-down exercises are essentially identical to chin- or pull-ups on an overhead bar.

As mentioned in the bent-over rowing section, some machines permit a pulling-in motion that is somewhere between a true lat pull-down and a horizontal rowing exercise. Muscle involvement is similar in all three movements, but there are some differences. For example, a pure horizontal (pulley) rowing motion strengthens the posterior deltoid but not the pec minor, while just the opposite is true for a lat pull-down.

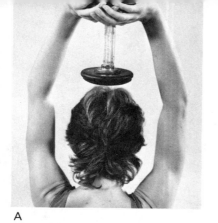
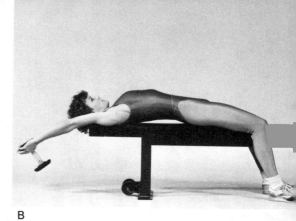

A   B

The straight-arm dumbbell pullover
The correct method for holding the dumbbell in the straight-arm pullover (A). From a

Pullover

Active Joints: Shoulder, shoulder girdle

Prime Movers: Pectoralis major and minor, latissimus dorsi, posterior deltoid

Equipment: Barbell, dumbbell, or machine

Proper Execution: You perform this exercise lying supine on a flat bench, holding either a barbell or dumbbell in your hands.

One method of doing the pullover is to keep your arms straight. If you use a barbell, use a pronated grip, hands about shoulder width apart or slightly less. Start by holding the bar at arms' length over your chest, identical to the starting position for the bench press except for the narrower grip. While keeping your arms straight, *slowly* lower the bar over and past your head until your arms are parallel to the floor. Immediately reverse the movement and slowly bring the bar back to the starting position. Breathe in deeply while lowering the bar, and exhale as you near the starting position on return. If you use a dumbbell rather than a barbell, keep the movement the same but hold the dumbbell with

The bent-arm pullover
The barbell is raised from below and behind the head to a position over the chest.

A   B

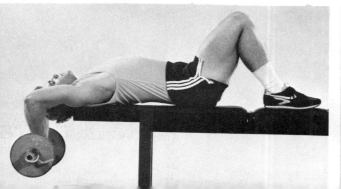
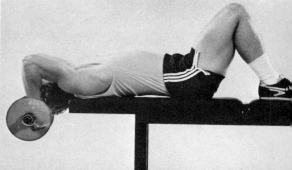

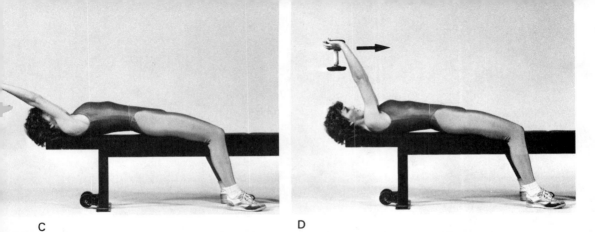

C   D

supine position, with the weight behind the head and arms straight (B), pull the weight over the body (C) to a final position directly over the chest (D), as shown with arrow.

cupped hands. The straight-arm pullover must be done with relatively light weights, and is often considered a breathing movement to be done after heavier exercises, such as the squat, to try to increase lung volume and expand the rib cage. But it will certainly help to strengthen the muscles it activates (also see bent-arm pullover below) and can even help strengthen the elbow joint after injury when elbow movement is painful or undesirable. The elbow strengthening effect is mainly on connective tissues that are stressed when the weight is held with straight arms parallel to the floor.

A second method of performing the pullover is identical to that described above except that the arms are bent at the elbow joints. The elbow is flexed and held fixed primarily by isometric contraction of the triceps muscle, and the elbow angle should not change during any phase of the pullover. As with the straight-arm pullover, you can use a barbell or a dumbbell. If you use a barbell, narrow your grip, placing hands about three inches apart. The weight used in a bent-arm pullover can be considerably heavier than with the straight-arm method due to improved leverage, and you will develop strength in the prime movers faster than in the straight-arm pullover. Study the illustrations on pages 100–101 to ensure that you use the correct techniques.

C   D

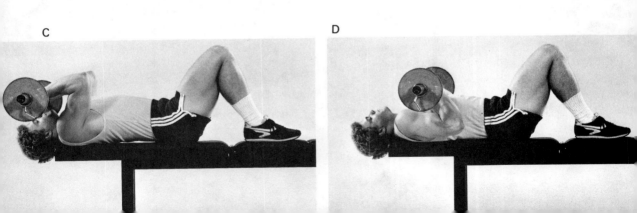

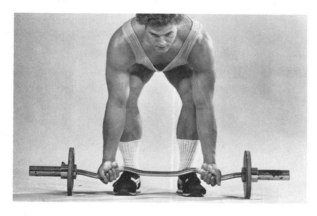

For many strength trainees, pullovers and other arm and shoulder exercises feel more comfortable with an e-z curl bar.

Like the other exercises previously discussed, pullovers have both a concentric and an eccentric muscle contraction phase. As the resistance is lowered, the prime movers slowly yield to the pull of gravity on the weight and thus lengthen. During the upward return to the starting position, the same muscles must generate enough tension to overcome the pull of gravity and shorten.

Some of you may feel more comfortable using an "e-z curl bar" rather than a normal barbell for bent-arm pullovers. This is because an e-z curl bar permits you to use a partially supinated grip rather than a completely pronated grip (if you've forgotten these hand positions, review page 19). This specially shaped bar is frequently used in various arm exercises and is discussed again in the Assistance Exercises section later in this chapter (also see the illustrations on pages 133 and 135). If you do not have access to an e-z curl bar and don't like the feel of doing pullovers with a standard bar, I'd recommend using a dumbbell.

Pullover machines
Most offer resistance through the entire range of motion.

A

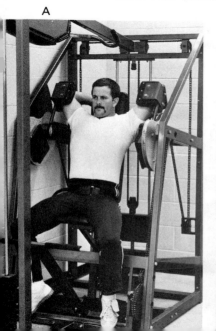

B

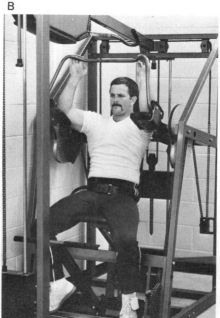

C

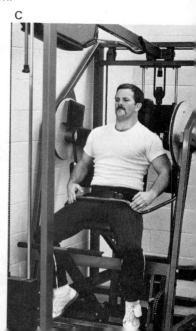

Some machines permit a pullover motion, such as the Nautilus device shown on page 102. When designed properly, pullover machines have the advantage of offering resistance through the full range of motion. The resistance offered by free weights during a pullover decreases toward the end of the movement range over the chest, since you're no longer moving the weight upward against gravity.

TORSO EXERCISES

The "pushing" and "pulling" exercises discussed above develop arm and shoulder muscles, as well as a number of upper back and chest muscles. Exercises discussed in this section work the abdominal and middle and lower back muscles that link the powerful leg and hip musculature to the upper body musculature. This torso region is very important for overall body strengthening and should never be the weakest link in the body chain. It is responsible for transferring muscle forces from upper-body to lower-body parts, and vice versa, as well as stabilizing and controlling movements of the spinal column.

Hyperextension

Active Joints: Intervertebral (joints in the spinal column)

Prime Movers: Spinal erectors

Equipment: Bench or floor, weight plates

Proper Execution: You can perform this exercise on a specially designed bench (see pages 104–105) or on a high flat bench or table with some padding at your hip and someone to hold down your legs. The edge of the padded bench or table should cross just below the tops of your pelvic bones (iliac crests) as you lie face down on it. From the starting position—spine fully flexed and head near the floor—lift your head and torso until they are slightly more than parallel with the floor. This is simply an extension and slight hyperextension of the spinal column due to concentric contraction of your spinal erector muscles. Then slowly reverse the motion, which results in another flexion of your spine controlled by eccentric contraction of the same muscles. Be sure you do the upward extension and slight hyperextension slowly to avoid a forced overextension of your spine at the upper end of the movement due to the momentum of your torso and head.

Hyperextensions

The hyperextension on a typical special-purpose bench
Note the position of the head and spine in (C)—only slightly more than parallel with the floor. Movements up and down should be slow.

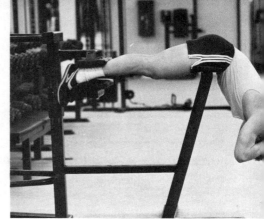

A

If you're a beginner, you should first try to perform an easier version of this exercise by lying face down on the floor, arms straight at your sides or hands clasped behind your head (see illustrations), and trying to raise your head, chest and shoulders slowly off the ground by contracting your lower back muscles (spinal erectors). This method limits the range of motion relative to a bench hyperextension, but it is a good way to start strengthening the spinal erectors. You can "graduate" to bench hyperextensions after a few weeks or months, whenever you're strong enough to do them properly.

As you continue to strengthen your lower back, you can also increase the resistance by holding weight plates behind your head.

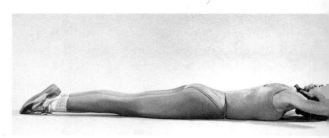

A

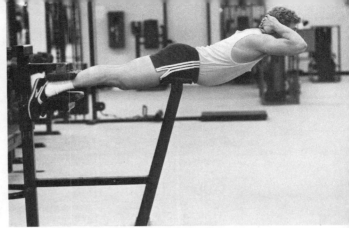

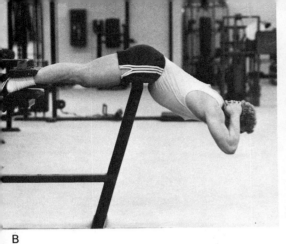

B

C

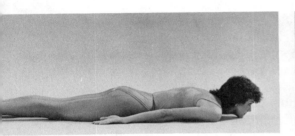

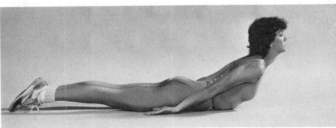

A

B

The hyperextension performed on the floor—hands at side
This is a good exercise to begin strengthening the spinal erector muscles.

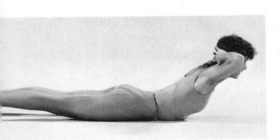

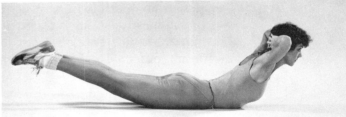

B

C

The hyperextension performed on the floor—hands behind head
This is the more strenuous version of the floor hyperextension. As your spinal erectors strengthen, try lifting both your head and your legs simultaneously (C).

Good Morning

Active Joints: Hip, intervertebral

Prime Movers: Hamstrings, gluteals, spinal erectors

Equipment: Barbell

Proper Execution: This is really a bending over movement similar to the one you might do to stretch and touch your toes in the morning. Hold a barbell firmly on your shoulders behind your head, keep your knees straight (fully extended) or slightly flexed, and lean forward slowly by flexing at the hip. You can do this exercise with either a straight back or flexed (rounded) back as shown in the illustrations. With a straight back, your spinal erectors are worked isometrically while your hamstrings and gluteals control hip flexion via an eccentric contraction. Return slowly to the starting upright position, using a concentric contraction of your hamstrings and gluteals. If you let your back round while leaning forward, your spinal erectors will be worked dynamically, contracting eccentrically with the downward movement and concentrically during the return movement. If you keep your knees slightly flexed, you will feel less pull across the back of your knees and you can use more weight on the barbell. I always recommend the bent-knee method for beginners. Likewise, with a straight back you'll be able to use more weight than with a rounded back. No matter which combination of knee and back conditions you choose for the "good morning" exercise, always do the movement slowly. Start with very light weight and increase it only very gradually over a period of weeks and months. It is important to strengthen your lower back, but if you're not careful and overdo it, you could suffer a back injury.

Good Morning

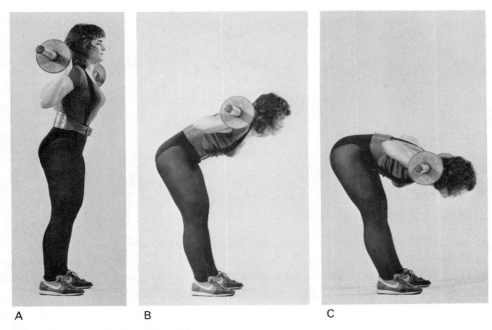

A   B   C

"Good morning"—legs straight
The movement down and up is slow.

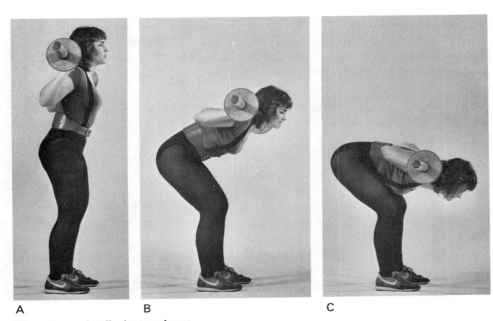

A   B   C

"Good morning"—knees bent
The bent-knee position should remain constant through the full range of motion. The movement down and up is done slowly.

Stiff Leg Deadlift

Active Joints: Hip, intervertebral

Prime Movers: Hamstrings, gluteals, spinal erectors

Equipment: Barbell or dumbbells

Proper Execution: You do this exercise while standing, using a pronated grip and holding a barbell about shoulders' width between your index fingers, arms hanging straight down. The movement and its variations, with or without back and knee flexion, and the muscles used are identical to the "good morning" exercise described above except for the way you hold the barbell. When you bend over to lower the bar, keep it as close to your legs as possible, and lower it slowly. Since the weight plates on the barbell limit range of motion when they reach the floor, some advanced trainees stand on a two- to four-inch block to permit the bar to be lowered to toe level (see page 125). The upward movement to return to the starting position should also be slow, and the bar should again be kept close to your legs. As with the "good morning" exercise, start doing this movement using very light weights and increase them gradually. You may also perform this exercise using dumbbells.

The Stiff-Leg Deadlift

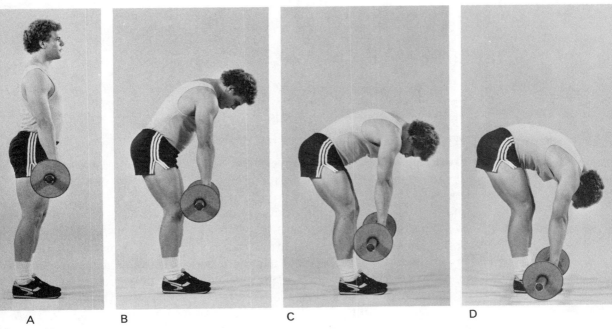

A   B   C   D

The stiff-leg deadlift—bent knees, rounded back
The movement down and up is slow and the bar should be kept close to the body
at all times.

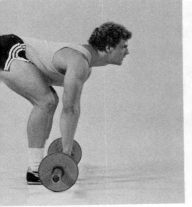
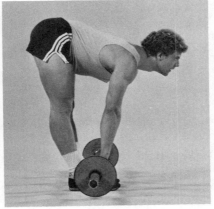
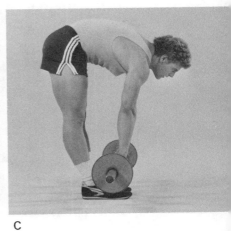

A   B   C

The stiff-leg deadlift—variations
Bent knees, straight back (A) Straight knees, straight back (B) Straight knees, rounded back (C)

ABDOMINAL EXERCISES

The Sit-Up and the Leg Lift

Active Joints: Intervertebral, hip

Prime Movers: Abdominals, hip flexors(?)

Equipment: Floor or "Ab" bench, weight plates

Proper Execution: The sit-up and the leg raise are familiar to almost everyone, and often are used for abdominal exercise. However, if you look closely at the movement sequences in the pictures of these exercises on pages 111 through 113, you'll see that extensive hip flexion (movement of the thighs toward the torso, or torso toward the thighs) occurs in both. The section on spinal column movement in Chapter 1 noted that the abdominal muscles run from the anterior pelvis to the lower rib cage, and that their contraction causes spinal flexion. The abdominals do not cross the hip joint, so they can't control or aid hip flexion. The section in Chapter 1 on hip movement lists the rectus femoris and iliopsoas as prime movers for hip flexion. Thus, the full sit-up shown in the illustration requires substantial use of the hip flexors. The abdominals are active concentrically in the movement from position (A) to (B), but then only isometrically to keep the spine flexed during the rest of the upward movement. Eccentric contraction of the hip flexors and, lastly, abdominals will control return to the starting position if the movement is done slowly.

Two possible problems exist with the sit-up as described above. First, it is inefficient to some extent since a major part of the exercise is under the control of hip flexors rather than the abdominal muscles. Second, and much more important, doing sit-ups can cause or aggravate lower back problems. How? The psoas major, strongest member of the iliopsoas muscle group, attaches to the lateral sides of the lumbar region of the spine (see page 22). This region of the spine naturally curves inward, and the pull of the psoas when it contracts tends to increase this curvature. That could eventually lead to or aggravate low back pain. This doesn't mean that the sit-up is a bad exercise. It means that the sit-up does not emphasize abdominal work as completely as we might think, and that doing sit-ups over long periods (especially while holding a weight plate behind the head or doing sit-ups on an incline) may contribute to low back pain. Of course, many of us with low back pain do sit-ups to strengthen the abdominals, which help maintain a level pelvic position and thereby reduce inward lumbar curvature. But for some people, doing sit-ups may actually aggravate the problem! The answer to this apparent dilemma is (1) not to worry if you are using sit-ups and have no low back problems or (2) change to exercises that work the abdominals but not the hip flexors.

If your choice is (1), be sure to do your sit-ups with bent knees. This increases the lever arm for psoas pull, and thus reduces the force needed to produce the required hip movement. If you choose (2), you should perhaps do only slow, partial sit-ups, often known as "trunk curls," or, do a trunk curl with your lower legs on a bench or chair to prevent hip flexion. Whenever you add twisting movements, such as left elbow toward right knee and vice versa, to a sit-up or a trunk curl, the external and internal oblique muscles of your abdominals are worked more extensively.

The leg raise exercise primarily involves hip flexion, with the abdominals used mainly in isometric contraction to stabilize the pelvis, on which some hip flexors pull. Again, if you use this exercise and have no low back problems, everything is fine. But remember the limited abdominal work involved and the extensive hip flexor action.

Bodybuilders often use a leg curl machine as illustrated to work the lower region of the rectus abdominus. Obviously, this movement primarily involves hip and knee flexion, but many individuals use it successfully. If it works for you, okay, but remember the possible connection with low back problems due to the strong hip flexion required. I should point out that the action of pulling the knees into the chest requires the pelvis to tilt upward—a movement caused by contraction of the lower section of the abdominal muscles. This short-range motion, by itself, is an excellent means of strengthening the lower abs.

The typical bent-knee sit-up
Note the initial spinal flexion (A) to (B), followed by hip flexion (B) to (C), making the bent-knee sit-up less than efficient for strengthening the abdominal muscles.

A

B

C

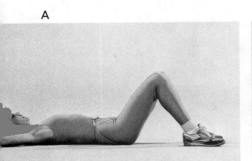
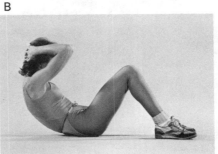
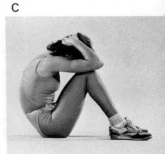

Other Abdominal and Hip Exercises

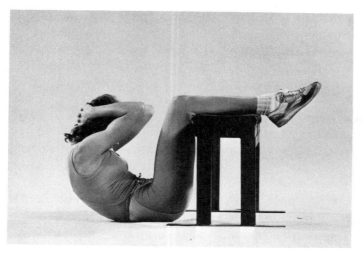

The partial sit-up, or trunk curl
Doing only partial sit-ups, or trunk curls, with or without
a bench to prevent hip flexion, helps work the abdominal muscles more efficiently.

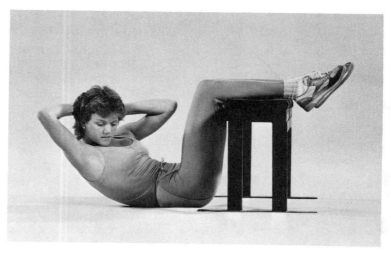

The twisting trunk curl
Twisting trunk curls exercise the oblique abdominal muscles.

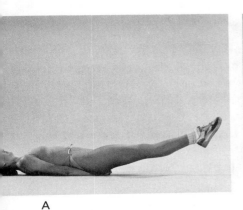
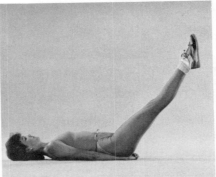
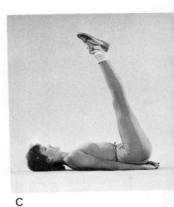

A   B   C

The leg raise
Note that only the hip joint moves (flexion of the hip).

Some trainees use the leg curl machine as an abdominal exerciser even though doing so strengthens primarily the hip flexors. The lower abdominals are worked mostly isometrically.

A   B

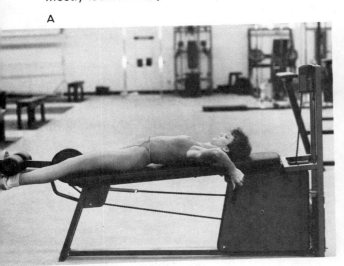
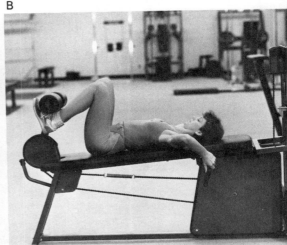

"TOTAL BODY" EXERCISES

Some lifting exercises involve so many joints and muscles of the body that they can aptly be called "total body" exercises. A barbell or dumbbells are the only equipment needed for these exercises; in fact, this is one reason the "total body" is so completely involved—*no* machine is involved to help do the work these exercises require. Many trainees avoid these exercises because they are strenuous and more difficult to learn than most of the other strength exercises. But progress depends on the effort you invest. If you want to train like the top strength athletes, you should try to incorporate at least some of the following primary exercises into your program.

The Squat

Proper Execution: To perform the most common method of squats—which are often called deep knee bends—hold a barbell firmly on your shoulders, behind your neck. The barbell is usually lifted from a rack or stand, but may be taken from two partners who lift it by the bar ends to your shoulders. Your feet should be about shoulder-width apart or slightly wider, with the toes straight ahead or pointing slightly outward. You'll probably have to experiment a little with foot position to find what's most comfortable for you.

In a slow, controlled manner, squat until your thighs are parallel with the ground. During the slow descent, keep your back tight and slightly arched, your chest out, your eyes focused straight ahead, and your feet flat on the floor. The calfs, quadriceps, hamstrings, and gluteals control descent via eccentric contractions. The torso retains rigidity via isometric contraction of the abdominals, spinal erectors, and shoulder girdle muscles, while the bar is held in place by shoulder and arm musculature. During the movement, avoid (1) rounding your

The parallel squat
The descent is slow, the back tight and slightly arched. The lowest position (C) occurs when the thighs are parallel to the ground.

A

B

C

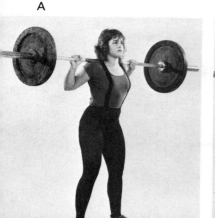
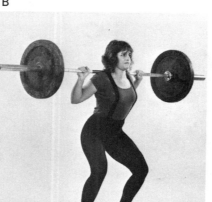
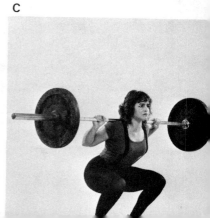

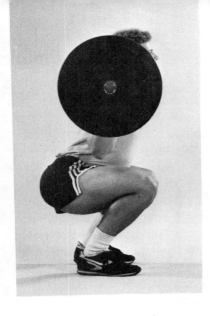

Side view, correct lowest position during the parallel squat
The thighs are parallel to the ground, the knees only slightly forward of the toes, and the forward lean of the torso is minimal.

back, (2) leaning too far forward at the hip, (3) letting your knees move too far forward, well in front of your toes, (4) squatting too deep, and (5) bouncing up from the "bottom" position. Reasons: (1) It is much easier with respect to muscular effort to support a barbell on your shoulders when your back is straight. (2) Leaning forward turns the squat into a modified "good morning" exercise, putting excess stress on your back, and does not emphasize use of your leg and hip muscles. (3) If your knees move too far forward, the amount of knee flexion is excessive, and unnecessarily large joint forces develop. (4) Squatting too low and (5) bouncing upward also create excessively large joint forces and are two of the main reasons squats have a bad reputation as a cause of knee problems.

While rising from the squat to the upright standing position, keep your body's forward torso lean as slight as possible. You can rise out of the squat faster than you lowered into it, but try to maintain proper body positions throughout the motion (study the illustrations!). Hip and leg muscles are prime movers for the upward concentric phase of the lift. Concentrate on forcing your hips forward while keeping your back arched during the ascent to help you maintain correct body position.

You can do the same squatting movement while holding a barbell across your shoulders in *front* of your neck. This is called a *front squat,* and it requires a rigorously vertical torso position to minimize the barbell's tendency to slide forward off your shoulders. In general, keeping the torso vertical for both front and back squats is important, since less forward torso lean reduces the muscular forces required in the low back area. Front squats work the lower quadriceps more extensively than standard "back" squats.

You may find it difficult to squat using either of the above techniques because you lack flexibility, particularly in your ankles. An aid in this situation is to place small weight plates, or a one- to two-inch thick board, under your heels while squatting. Either should help you maintain balance and proper form through each phase of the exercise. Think of this only as a temporary aid though, until the flexibility of your ankles, knees, and hips increase and you can stop using the heel elevation.

Many people cheat and do only partial squats, never lowering their thighs enough to be parallel to the ground. I discourage this type of squatting, since it limits the range of motion and muscle action and decreases the work done. Partial squats can be helpful if you are trying to "get the feel" of a heavier weight before doing a full squat with it or if you are just learning the movement and getting used to the balance and body positions. Also, if for some reason such as an injury you can't do a full squat, then "partials" can be better than no squats at all (in this situation, also consider leg presses or lunges).

You should always be careful and use common sense when doing squats. If at all possible, have a spotter stand behind you to help support or lift the weight if you lose your balance or cannot get up from the lower squat position. A spotter standing at each end of the bar is safer yet. If you don't have someone to spot you, there are various types of safety racks you can use that permit total freedom of movement when doing squats and other barbell exercises but make it impossible for you to drop the weight on yourself or get pinned under it (one type is shown in the illustrations). You can easily build such a safety rack by drilling appropriate sized holes in two-by-six-inch wooden beams and using old pipe sections for the variable height support pins. If you're not the do-it-yourself type, you can buy any of a variety of safety racks from barbell and exercise equipment companies at a reasonable price. Check the ads found in some weightlifting magazines for leads on such products. If you're lifting in a public gym, a safety rack should be available, so use it.

If the worst happens and you are squatting alone without a safety rack and lose your balance or cannot rise from the squat without dropping the weight, be prepared to protect yourself. Depending on your body position or which way you've lost your balance, you can duck your head and rapidly push the barbell over it onto the floor, or push the barbell backward while pushing yourself forward to jump away from it. In either case, the barbell or floor may be damaged but you'll be okay—and probably a little more careful in the future.

Squats may be done with less resistance—and with no need for a rack or spotters—by holding dumbbells in the hands. You can also do "hack" squats by standing in front of a barbell that is on the floor just behind your heels, squatting down to grasp the bar, and then rising and squatting repeatedly while holding the bar behind you.

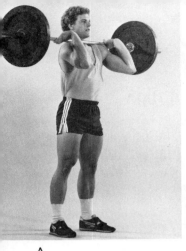
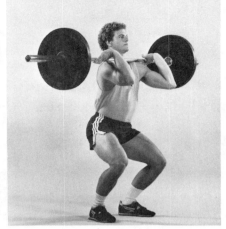
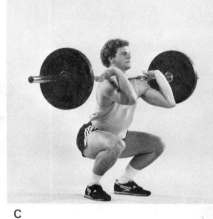

A   B   C

The front squat
Note that the bar is resting on the shoulders and is not fully supported on the hands. The elbows are held high and the torso remains relatively vertical through the full range of movement.

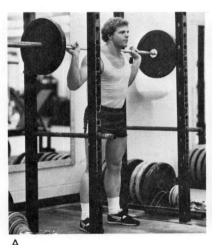
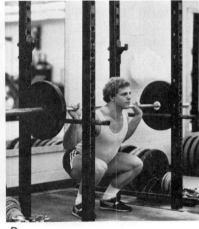

Squatting in a rack with variable-height safety pins eliminates the need for a spotter.

A   B

The hack squat
(A) shows the starting and finishing position. Return the weight from position (D) slowly to the floor.

A   B   C   D

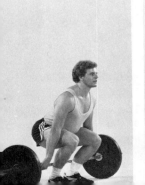
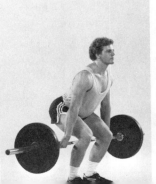
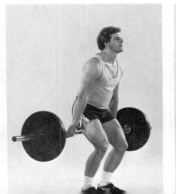
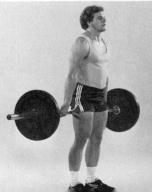

Pulling Movements: The Power Clean and High Pull

Pulling movements are lifting exercises in which you pull a barbell held in your hands upward from the floor, or an intermediate height, toward your shoulders. Pulls have certain similarities to the squat, just as "stiff leg" deadlifts have similarities with "good mornings." The most frequently used pulling exercises are the power clean and the high pull.

Proper Execution: At the start of the power clean, rest the barbell on the floor in front of you, close to your shins, so that the bar is over the front of your feet. Keep your back tight and slightly arched (as in the squat), and bend your knees and hips until you can grasp the bar (palms facing toward you) with straight arms and a shoulder-width grip. Your feet should also be about shoulder width apart, with your toes straight ahead or pointed slightly to the side. Study the following illustrations, and be aware that this starting position *will* feel uncomfortable at first.

You begin the lift by gradually extending your knees. The bar should move upward very close to your shins. Your torso angle with the horizontal should be nearly constant from "lift-off" until the bar clears your kneecaps. Don't let your hips rise faster than your shoulders. At this point, your balance on each foot should return to the ball of the foot, having moved from between the ball of your foot and arch at "lift-off" toward the heel as the bar reached knee level. Your hips move forward, toward the bar, during this balance shift, while your knees rebend slightly and shift forward under the bar. Simultaneously, your

The Power Clean

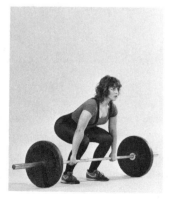

Starting position (A)

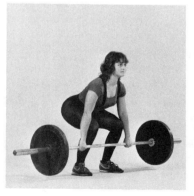

Just after "lift-off" (B)

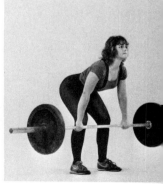

The end of the first pull as the bar reaches knee level (C)

torso extends at the hip to become almost vertical, but your shoulders should still be over the bar rather than behind it. From this shifted position (keep studying the illustrations) a very rapid explosive jump straight upward must occur via knee and hip extension, ankle plantar flexion, and "shrugging" of the shoulder girdle by violent trapezius contraction.

Up to this point in the movement, your arms should act like ropes attaching the bar to your shoulders. Only at the end of this straight upward jump do your arms begin to pull on the bar as your elbows flex and move upward and sideward. At this point, the bar is moving rapidly upward, and you must shift your body under it rapidly to catch the weight and complete the power clean.

Be sure to catch the weight on your shoulders and clavicles and *not* let it rest solely on your hands. To catch the bar properly, pull it as high as possible along your torso, and when you reach the so-called "top pull" position—on your toes with your knees and hips fully extended and elbows up and out to the side—rapidly rotate your elbows down under and then up in front of the bar as it touches your shoulders and clavicles. As your elbows rotate around the bar, you should bend (flex) your knees so that when the barbell lands on your shoulders, your knees can give slightly and act like shock absorbers to stop smoothly the downward motion of the bar by eccentric contraction of the quadriceps. Never catch the bar while your knees are fully extended since the bones could be jammed together (which will hurt!) from the force of the catch. Carefully return the barbell to the floor and reposition yourself for the next rep.

For a "high pull," pull the bar as high to your chest as possible, but then

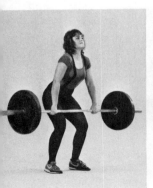
The finish of the shift and start of the second pull (D)

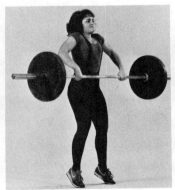
The finish of the second, or "top," pull position (E)

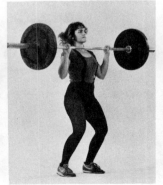
Moving under the bar by bending the knees and rotating the elbows under the bar (F)

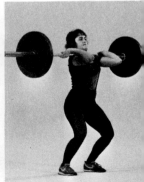
The finish, or catch (G)

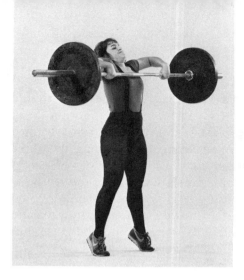

The high pull—clean grip position

From the maximum high-pull position (shown here) the bar is returned immediately to the floor. High pulls are often done with heavier weights, resulting in the bar reaching only waist height.

immediately return it to the floor. Do the "first pull" (lift-off to knee level) for either of these lifts at moderate speed, and try to maintain the proper body positions and a tight back throughout. Do the shift—also called the "scoop" or second knee bend—before the jump at moderate speed as well, but make the jump itself very fast and explosive. This jump or "second pull" is biomechanically similar in leg and hip action to a vertical jump and is very useful in developing jumping ability and explosiveness in athletes.

The Power Snatch

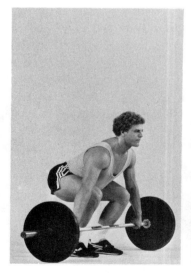

Starting position (A)

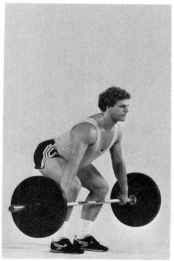

Just after "lift-off" (B)

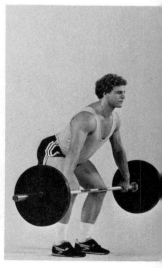

The end of the first pull as the bar reaches knee level (C)

The Power Snatch and Snatch Grip High Pull

Proper Execution: The power snatch and snatch high pull require almost identical pulling technique to the power clean and high pull explained above. The differences are that your hand grip spacing is much greater, that lighter weights are used, and that the goal of the power snatch is to catch the barbell overhead rather than at your shoulders. It is difficult to tell you exactly how wide a grip to use, but it will probably be at least 10 inches wider than your clean grip width. Because of the wider grip, your hips and shoulders will be closer to the ground in the starting or "lift-off" position. Use of the wide grip will permit you to catch the barbell overhead with straight arms after pulling it to a lower height than you would need if you used a narrower (clean width) grip. You perform the pull for a snatch lift just as you would for the power clean, but with the following differences: From the top pull position (hands with the wider grip) and with the lighter barbell moving faster than in a clean, bend your knees slightly, rapidly rotate your elbows under the bar as it passes your head and push the bar upward to catch it overhead with your arms straight. To stop your knee bend as you catch the barbell overhead, strongly contract your quadriceps.

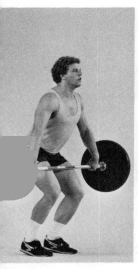

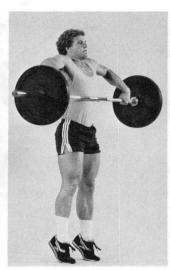

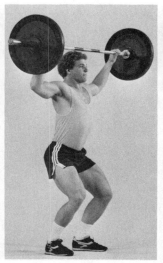

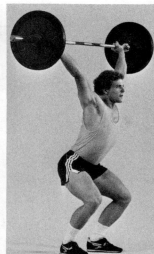

The finish of the shift and start of the second pull (D)

The finish of the second, or "top," pull position (E)

Moving under the bar by bending the knees, rotating the elbows under the bar and pushing the arms up (F)

The finish, or catch (G)

Then, carefully return the barbell to the floor and reposition yourself for the next rep.

The snatch grip high pull, like the clean grip high pull, ends when the bar reaches its highest point at the end of the second pull (top pull position) and is then immediately returned to the floor. With the wide grip and relatively lighter weight, you may, in the snatch grip high pull, be able to pull the bar above your chest or to chin level.

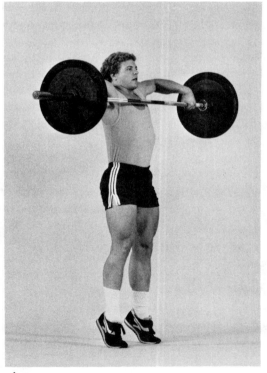 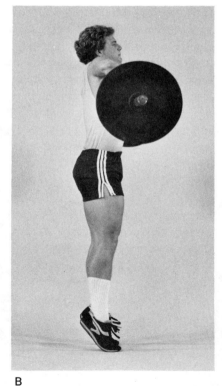

A   B

The high pull—snatch grip position
Notice in both (A) and (B) the vertical position of the body, the closeness of the bar to the body, and how the elbows are up and pointing out to the side.

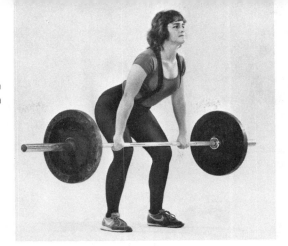

Starting position for a clean from knee level rather than from the floor

Partial Pulls and Pulling Variations

A common variation of the pulling movements discussed above is to do them from just above knee level rather than from the floor, starting either with the bar held in your hands against your thighs, or with the weights initially supported on boxes or by a rack. These methods require only the fast second pull, but they are useful for developing speed and explosiveness in your leg and hip muscles. These partial pulling movements are also useful as a teaching aid because they allow you to concentrate your attention on one part of the total pulling motion at a time. The first pull—lift-off to knee height—can also be practiced separately, as can the shift or transition from first to second pull (see illustrations).

High pull from a rack support
Boxes may also be used to support the weights at the starting height desired.

A

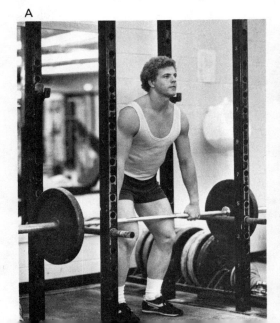

B

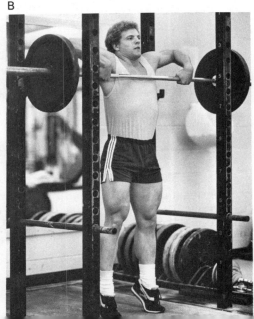

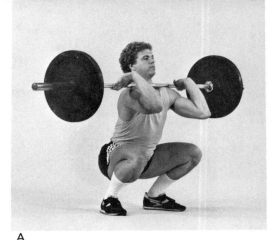

A

Competitive squat positions to catch the weight
The deep-squat clean position (A) and the squat snatch position (B) are both used in competitive weightlift-ing.

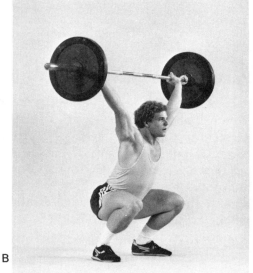

B

If your knees bend too much when you catch a power clean, the weight may force you into a low front squat position and the lift becomes a squat clean, as used in competitive Olympic-style weightlifting. This should not happen if you choose reasonable weights. The same considerations apply to the power snatch versus squat snatch, the only differences being that with a snatch you use a wider hand grip and catch the weight at arms' length overhead rather than at the shoulders as in the clean.

In addition to cleans or snatches from above knee level and "high-pulls" done with either a snatch or clean width grip, other variations of basic pulling exercises include the pull and shrug, pull to knee level, and pull from elevation. The pull and shrug (also see "shoulder shrug" on page 140) is identical to the high pull except that the arms bend very little after the second pull and trapezius "shrug." As a result, the bar does not rise much higher than the waist. Heavier weights are generally used in this exercise than in the high pull or power clean or snatch. Pulls to knee level are just the first pull of the clean or

The pull and shrug

Pull the bar from the floor just as you would for a power clean (page 118). But rather than lifting the bar to your chest, finish the exercise by raising the bar with a rapid upward shrug of the shoulders with little or no elbow bend, as shown. Heavier weights can be used because of the more limited range of motion.

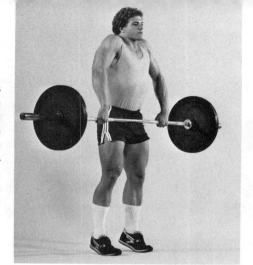

snatch, the bar being lifted only to the knees. Again, a relatively heavy weight can be used. If you're using this partial movement to learn how to pull properly, however, keep the weight light. Finally, you can do any of the pulling movements from the floor while standing on wooden boards or some other type of elevation. This brings the starting position of the bar closer to the feet and increases the range of motion during the lift. The same idea was discussed in the section on the stiff leg deadlift. Pulls from elevation are strenuous for the leg, hip, and low back area and should not be done by beginners. Remember, all the partial or modified pulling movements discussed above can be done with either a clean or a snatch width grip.

The high pull from elevation

Standing on a board or similar platform increases the range of motion during any type of pull.

A

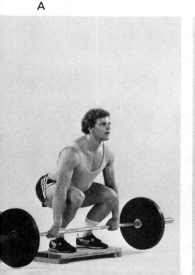

B

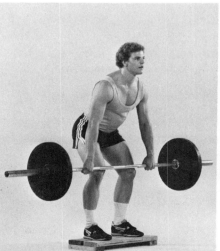

C

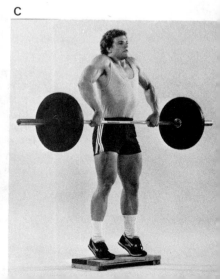

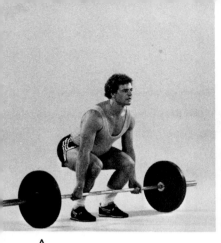
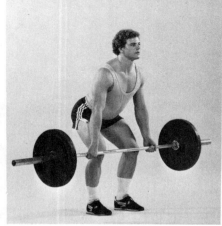
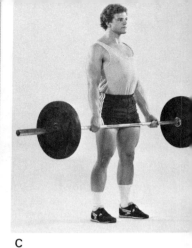

A   B   C

The deadlift
This movement is slow and the bar is lifted no higher than mid-thigh level. Note the opposing hand positions, which help maintain grip when lifting heavy weights during this exercise.

The Deadlift

Proper Execution: For some of you, the slower deadlift may be more suitable in your program than pulls since it's easier to do. This lift is similar to the pull and shrug discussed above, except that its finish occurs when your knees and hips are fully extended, your torso is vertical, and the bar is at mid-thigh level with your arms straight and shoulders back. This movement is done more slowly than any of the other pulling lifts, but otherwise it works the leg, hip, and back muscles in a similar manner. You can shrug your shoulders (contract your trapezius muscles) at the end of the deadlift, making the overall movement a slow version of the pull and shrug. Also, you'll find you can handle rather heavy weights in the deadlift, but be sure to increase the weight gradually if you're a beginner.

A

The push press
Start with the bar at the shoulders (A), dip at the knees and hips slightly (B), and "thrust" the bar upward, using leg and hip drive, to about the level of the top of the head (C). Keep the bar moving by pressing it upward to arm's length in one continuous motion (D).

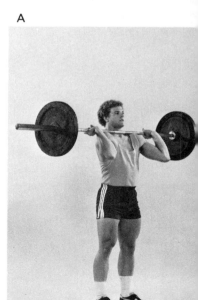

With the above introduction to the important pulling lifts—and the illustrations—you can begin to learn one or more of them and make them a productive part of your program. *Practice with light weights* and, if need be, seek additional instruction from other references or knowledgeable strength coaches and fitness instructors.

Shoulder to Overhead Lifts

The remaining three total body lifts, discussed below, require that you lift a barbell from your shoulders to arms' length overhead. At first glance, you may wonder why these movements were not covered in the "upper body pushing exercises" section. The reason is that the leg and hip musculature is primarily or totally responsible for propelling the weight overhead, with many other muscles involved in a stabilizing or support capacity. If you practice any of these lifts, you'll find that they do involve the total body.

Push Press

Proper Execution: This exercise is similar to an overhead press done from the standing position (review its technique on pages 88–90). At the start, however, with the barbell held firmly at your shoulders, you now dip quickly and only slightly at the knees and hips and immediately thrust the bar straight upward with rapid knee and hip extension, but only forcefully enough to "throw" the bar to about the level of the top of your head. Keep the bar moving upward by pressing it straight up to arms' length overhead, as you would finish a regular overhead press. The advantages of this exercise over the standing press are: (1)

B

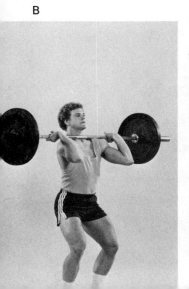

C

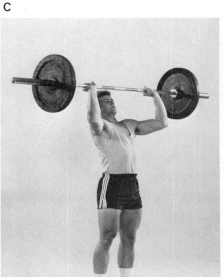

D

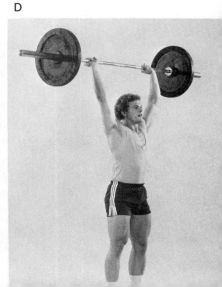

more weight can be lifted, (2) the leg and hip muscles are used, and in an explosive manner (although the range of motion is limited), and (3) more total muscle groups are used and at a faster speed of contraction. To begin the exercise, either "clean" the barbell from the floor to the shoulders or take it from stands or a rack. If you prefer, use dumbbells, letting the weights rest partly on your shoulders at the start.

Push Jerk

Proper Execution: This movement is similar to the push press, except that the knee and hip dip at the start is a little deeper and the knee and hip thrust to drive the barbell upward is much more forceful (similar to the jump phase or second pull of a power clean). This thrust actually throws, or "jerks," the barbell to arms' length overhead. You don't have to press it up. But you should think of a pressing action toward the end of the movement to hold the bar steady overhead, or to finish the movement if the leg thrust was not powerful enough to propel the bar all the way up to arms' length overhead. You can use a relatively heavy weight in this exercise, but you must keep your torso very tight, and you must hold the bar firmly at your shoulders during the dip and initial upward drive. Your dip must be straight downward with no forward torso lean, and your upward thrust must be straight up with no forward incline, or else the bar will be thrown forward, making it very difficult to support. Always catch the weight overhead with your knees bent. This is a very productive exercise for developing explosive strength (power) in the leg and hip musculature.

A

B

C

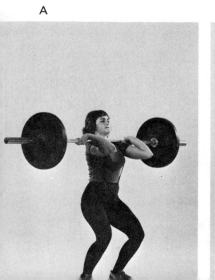
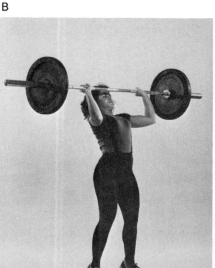
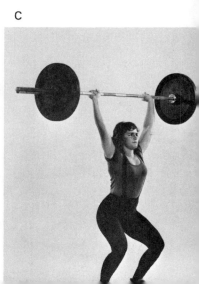

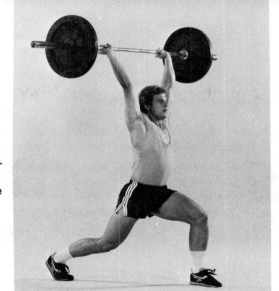

Catching the barbell in a split position after jerking it overhead
The start and thrust phases are the same as in the push jerk.

Split Jerk

Proper Execution: The split jerk is performed the same way as the push jerk, except for the position of the feet while the arms are catching the bar overhead. At the end of the rapid and forceful knee and hip thrust to "throw" the barbell upward—that is, as it moves toward arms' length overhead—rapidly shift one foot forward and one backward. Which foot moves front and which back is a matter of preference, but both feet should touch the ground at the same time. From this split position with the weight overhead, first push backward with the front foot and step back, then push forward with the back foot and step forward so that the feet are side by side.

D

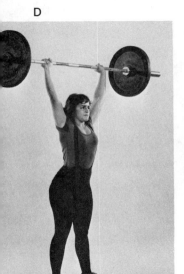

The push jerk
The start is similar to the push press, but the legs and hips are more deeply flexed (A). Explosive leg and hip drive (B) propels the barbell to arm's length (C) without any pressing phase. The catch always occurs with bent knees, which straighten for final support (D).

ASSISTANCE EXERCISES

Assistance exercises tend to isolate and develop smaller muscles and muscle groups. They are of less overall importance to a total body strengthening program than are the primary exercises discussed previously, due to the limited effects they produce. They can be productive, however, in contributing to specific goals, such as neck strength for a wrestler or a football player, or grip strength for a tennis player. Assistance movements may also be valuable in the rehabilitation of an injured joint or muscle.

Elbow Curl

Active Joint: Elbow

Prime Movers: Elbow flexor muscles

Equipment: Barbell, dumbbell, e-z curl bar, or machine

Proper Execution: This exercise involves only a flexion movement at the elbow, controlled by concentric contraction of the elbow flexors. You can use a barbell, dumbbells, pulley devices, or various specialized machines to perform elbow curls from either a standing or a seated position. A slow eccentric contraction of the four elbow flexors should be used to return the resistance to the starting position. Your elbow joint should be the only joint that moves during this exercise; do not swing or rotate your torso to lift heavier weights; that's cheating. You can stand against a wall or sit with a back support to avoid torso involvement, but you should use the fullest possible range of elbow-joint flexion and extension during curls.

Most trainees use a palms-up, shoulder-width grip with a barbell. But you can also use a pronated (palms-down) grip to involve the muscles on the

A

The standing barbell curl
The elbows stay fixed at the sides; the torso should not lean backward.

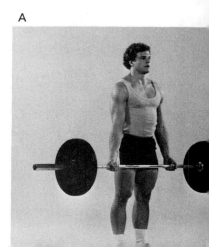

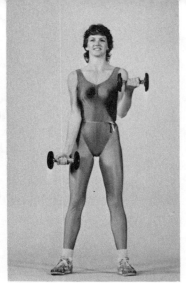

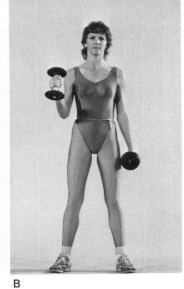

Elbow Curls

The standing alternate dumbbell curl
Dumbbell curls can be done using either a supinated (A) or partially pronated grip (B).

A

B

Barbell curl with reverse (pronated) grip

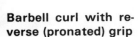

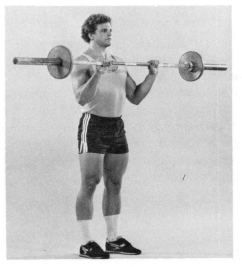

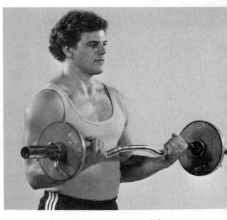

The curl with an e-z curl bar
The e-z curl permits a partially pronated grip.

B

C

D

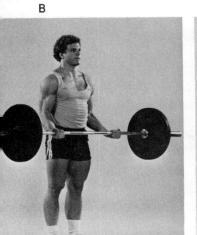

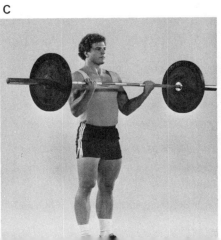

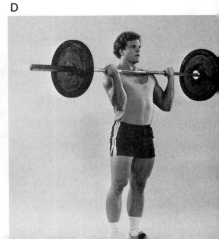

opposite side of the forearm and to work the elbow flexors with a different angle of pull. An e-z curl bar is a modified version of a normal bar with a bent gripping region. It permits a partly pronated grip for curling and several other exercises. You may find this type of grip very comfortable. It also provides a different angle of pull for the working muscles.

When you use dumbbells for curling, a variety of grip positions between fully pronated and supinated are possible, each resulting in a slightly different angle of pull on the elbow flexor muscles.

Triceps Extension

Active Joint: Elbow

Prime Mover: Triceps

Equipment: Barbell, dumbbell, pulley device, or machine

Proper Execution: This exercise also involves movement only at the elbow joint and can be done while seated or standing. You can use a barbell, holding it with a narrow hand grip, or a dumbbell, cupping your hands around one end. The movement starts with your arms fully extended overhead. Slowly lower the weight via eccentric contraction of the triceps until your elbows are fully flexed. From there, push the weight back to the starting position by concentrically contracting the triceps. Be sure to move only the elbow joints—no others!

You can also do elbow extension exercises using various pulley devices and other specialized machines.

A

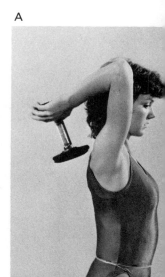

The dumbbell triceps extension
Cup one end of the dumbbell just as you would for a straight-arm dumbbell pullover (see page 100).

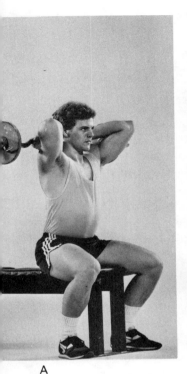 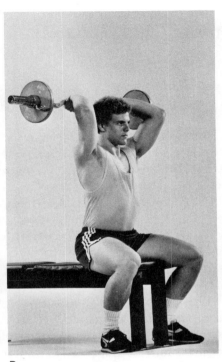 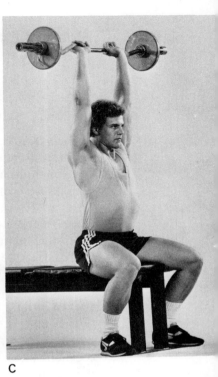

A   B   C

The triceps extension, or triceps press
This exercise can be done seated or standing, with a straight barbell or e-z curl bar (shown here).

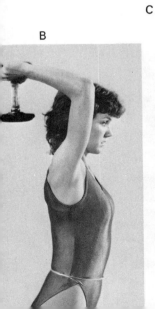 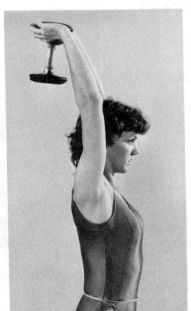

B   C

Forearm Exercises

Active Joints: Wrist, finger joints

Prime Movers: Wrist and finger flexors and extensors

Equipment: Barbell or dumbbell

Proper Execution: Every exercise done holding a barbell or dumbbell in your hands will improve grip and wrist strength, which are highly dependent on forearm musculature. In some situations you may wish to place additional emphasis on forearm strength. Various types of spring-loaded grip "squeezers" are available to develop your finger flexion strength, though an old tennis ball can be equally effective. Barbell and dumbbell wrist curl (palms up) and wrist extension (palms down) movements can be performed on a bench or table to emphasize different forearm muscles. To perform the curl or flexion movement, simply roll the bar from the fingertips up into a tight fist while your forearm(s) rest on the support, wrist(s) just over the edge. Wrist extensions are done while the bar is held with a firm, pronated grip, with the wrist(s) just over the edge of the support surface and fully flexed at the start. Extend your wrist(s) until hyperextended, then return to the starting position. Both the concentric and eccentric phases of these movements are important and should be done at slow to medium speed. A piece of a broomstick and a cord of some type can be used to make a "wrist roller." By tying a weight to one end of the cord and rolling the weight up and down, you can work your forearm muscles vigorously.

Three Basic Forearm Exercises

The barbell wrist curl

A

B

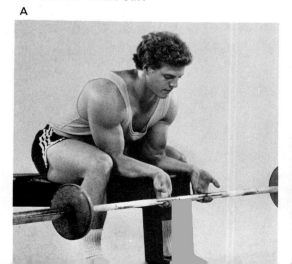
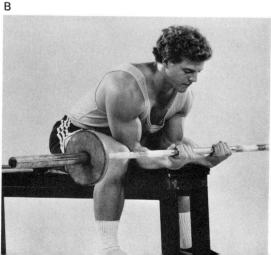

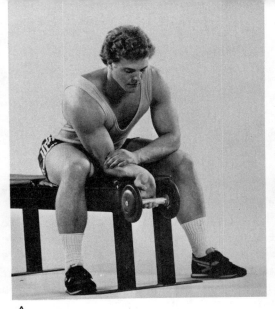
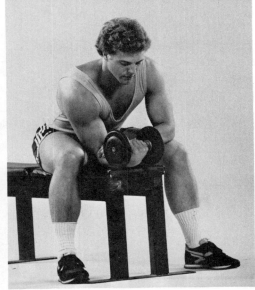

A   B

The dumbbell wrist curl

The wrist roller
Roll the weight both up and down.

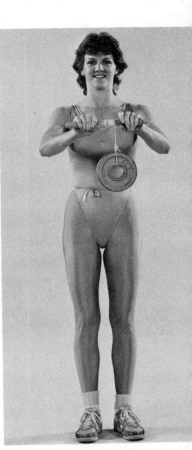

A   B

Neck Exercises

Active Joint: Intervertebral (cervical spine)

Prime Movers: Neck muscles

Equipment: Head strap, manual resistance

Proper Execution: Some sports, such as football, wrestling, and tumbling, require extra strengthening of the neck muscles. A number of machines are available for this purpose, but there are less expensive means for productive neck exercise. You can make or purchase a padded head strap to which weights are attached; wearing the strap, you move your head from side to side and front and back to lift the weights against gravity. Another simple method is to have a partner apply steady resistance, using a towel, while you perform various head movements. Neck bridging exercises, such as the wrestler's bridge, are dangerous, and I don't recommend them for anyone but advanced trainees. Whatever means you use to exercise your neck—if you feel you need it—start with very little neck work and very slowly increase the workload over a period of weeks and months. Keep in mind, too, that exercises that involve an upward swing of the shoulder girdle, such as upright rows, power cleans and shoulder shrugs (see below), also strengthen the muscles on the rear (posterior) side of the neck.

A

B

Manually applied resistance to neck movements using a towel and the help of a training partner For flexion strength, resistance is applied to the forehead (A, B). For lateral flexion strength, resistance is applied to the side of the head (C, D). For extension strength, resistance is applied to the back of the head. Resistance should be steady and all neck movements slow.

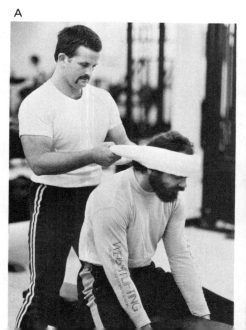
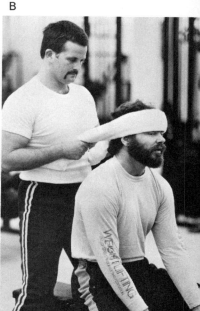

Neck-Strengthening Exercises

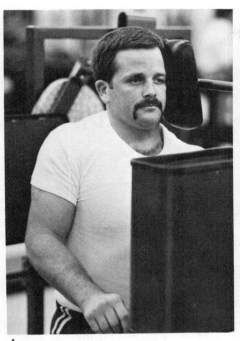

A

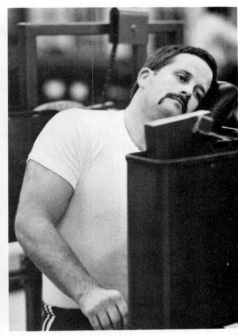

B

The Nautilus neck machine
With it, you can do lateral head movements, as shown, and anterior-posterior head movements against adjustable resistance.

C

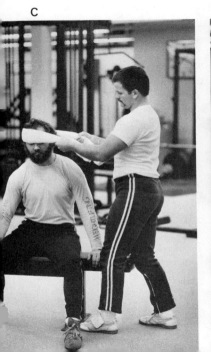

D

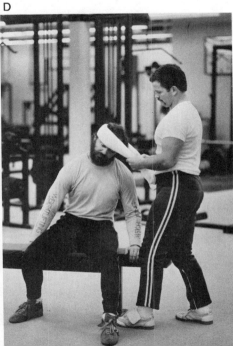

Lateral Raise

Active Joint: Shoulder

Prime Mover: Deltoid

Equipment: Dumbbell or weight plate

Proper Execution: Many of the exercises discussed previously work the deltoid muscle. A simple exercise called the lateral raise isolates and works all three parts of the deltoid together. Hold a weight plate or dumbbell in your hand, and with your elbow fully extended, lift (abduct) your arm to the side until it is horizontal with the floor. Then slowly return the weight to the starting position. The group of four small shoulder muscles called the rotator cuff are also worked with this exercise, making it valuable for rehabilitation after certain shoulder injuries. To emphasize the anterior (front) section of the deltoid, raise the dumbbells or a barbell in front of your body, starting at thigh-level and keeping your arms straight, by flexing the shoulder joints.

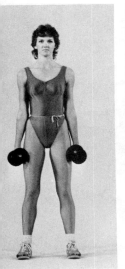 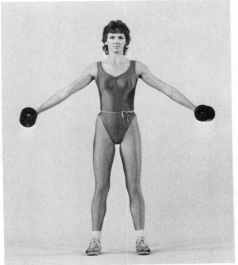 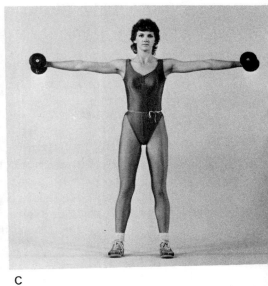

A B C

The lateral dumbbell raise
The movement up and down should be slow.

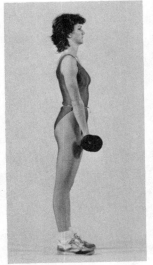 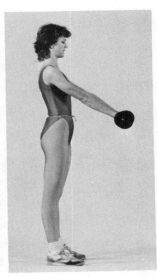 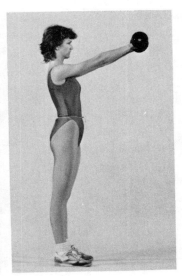

A B C

The forward dumbbell raise
This exercise works the anterior deltoid. The movement can also be done using a barbell.

Shoulder Shrug

Active Joint: Shoulder girdle

Prime Mover: Trapezius

Equipment: Barbell, dumbbells, or machine

Proper Execution: A number of the exercises previously described include a shrugging, or upward rotary motion of the shoulder girdle, which is controlled primarily by trapezius contraction. Shrugs, however, can be performed separately to isolate and emphasize the trapezius.

To perform a shrug, simply stand with a barbell or dumbbells in your hands and, while keeping your arms down, shrug your shoulders. You can do shrugs slowly or explosively. A few companies, such as Nautilus, manufacture a shoulder shrug machine.

Shoulder shrug with barbell

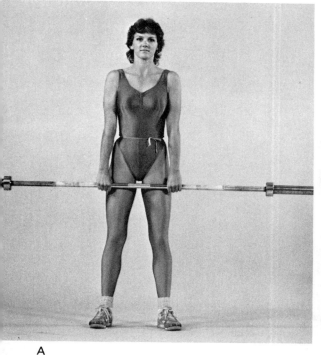 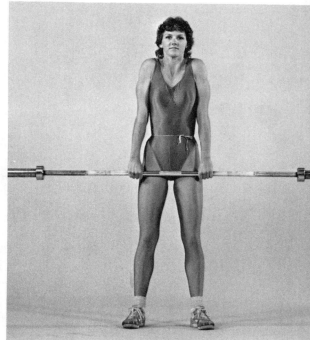

A   B

Shoulder shrug with dumbbells

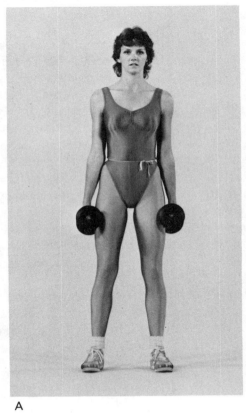

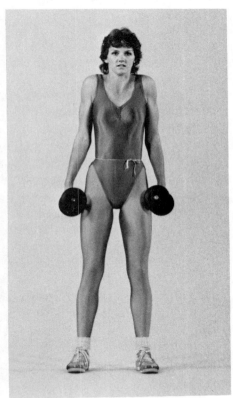

A

B

Dumbbell Flys

Active Joint: Shoulder

Prime Movers: Pectoralis major, anterior deltoid

Equipment: Dumbbells

Proper Execution: No, this exercise does not involve flying dumbbells. It does, however, primarily develop the pectoralis major and anterior deltoid. To perform dumbbell flys, start by lying on a flat bench with your arms holding dumbbells directly above your chest. Your elbows must be slightly flexed. With eccentric contraction of your pectoralis major and anterior deltoids, slowly lower the dumbbells to the side with a transverse abduction motion, so that the dumbbells feel as if they were pulling your chest apart at the sternum. Keep your elbows in a slightly flexed position throughout the movement, primarily via isometric contraction of your elbow flexors and extensors. The reverse movement to the starting position, a transverse adduction, is controlled by concentric contraction of the same prime movers. The bench press works these same muscles through a similar movement range, but also works other muscle groups such as the elbow extensors (triceps). And since it permits the use of much heavier weights, it should be considered the best chest, shoulder, and arm exercise.

Dumbbell flys are frequently used by bodybuilders as a supplemental chest and shoulder exercise, and they can be used to work these body areas if an elbow is injured. Some companies, such as Universal and Nautilus, provide machines that duplicate the dumbbell fly motion of the upper body, but while you are seated upright.

Dumbbell Flys

Elbow flexion remains constant throughout the movement, which should be slow both down and up.

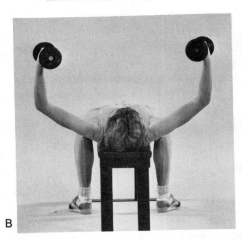

A

B

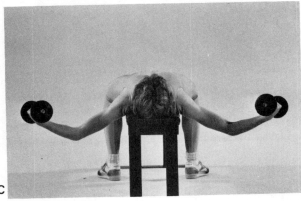

C

SUMMARY

The exercises described in this chapter are summarized in the following table. There are a number of other worthwhile exercises that could be discussed. But those described here represent the majority of important movements and offer a wide choice for your strength training program.

Strength Training Exercises

	Name	Prime Mover(s)	Synergists	Equipment
1.	Leg extensions	Quadriceps	—	Machine, iron boot
2.	Leg curls	Hamstrings	—	Machine, iron boot
3.	Calf raises	Gastroc, soleus	—	Machine, barbell
4.	Leg press	Quads, gluteals	Hamstrings	Machine, barbell
5.	Lunge	Quads, gluteals	Hamstrings	Barbell, dumbbells
6.	Squats	Total body	—	Barbell
7.	Bench press	Pectoralis major, deltoid	Triceps	Barbell, bench, machine, dumbbells
7a.	Push-ups	Pectoralis major	Triceps, deltoid	Floor
8.	Incline presses	Pectoralis major, deltoid	Triceps	Barbell, dumbbells, incline bench
9.	Overhead presses	Deltoid	Triceps, trapezius	Barbell, dumbbells
10.	Behind neck press	Deltoid	Triceps	Barbell
11.	Bent-over rowing	Latissimus dorsi	Deltoid, elbow flexors	Barbell, dumbbells, pulley
12.	Upright rowing	Trapezius	Deltoid, elbow flexors	Barbell, dumbbells, pulley
13.	Lat pull downs	Latissimus dorsi	Elbow flexors	Pulley
13a.	Wide grip chins	Latissimus dorsi	Elbow flexors	Horizontal bar
14.	Pullovers	Deltoid, pectoralis major	Serratus anterior	Barbell, dumbbells
15.	Hyperextension	Spinal erectors	—	Bench, floor
16.	Good mornings	Spinal erectors	Hamstrings	Barbell
17.	Stiff-leg deadlift	Spinal erectors	Hamstrings	Barbell, dumbbells
18.	Trunk curls	Abdominals	—	Floor

	Name	Prime Mover(s)	Synergists	Equipment
18a.	Situps	Iliopsoas	Abdominals	Floor
18b.	Leg raises	Iliopsoas	Abdominals	Floor
19.	Front squats	Total body	—	Barbell
20.	Cleans	Total body	—	Barbell
20a.	Snatches	Total body	—	Barbell
20b.	High pulls	Total body	—	Barbell
20c.	Dead lift	Total body	—	Barbell
21.	Push press	Total body	—	Barbell
22.	Push jerk	Total body	—	Barbell
23.	Split jerk	Total body	—	Barbell
24.	Curls	Elbow flexors	Forearm muscles	Barbell, dumbbells, pulley, machines
25.	Tricep extensions	Triceps	—	Barbell, dumbbells, pulley
26.	Wrist curls	Forearm muscles	—	Barbell, dumbbells
26a.	Wrist extensions	Forearm muscles	—	Barbell, dumbbells
26b.	Wrist roller	Forearm muscles	—	Roller and cord
26c.	Grip squeezes	Forearm muscles	—	Tennis ball
27.	Neck movements	Neck muscles	—	Head strap, machine, assistant and towel
28.	Lateral raises	Deltoid	—	Dumbbells
29.	Shoulder shrug	Trapezius	—	Barbell, dumbbells, machine
30.	Dumbbell flys	Pectoralis major	Deltoid	Dumbbells

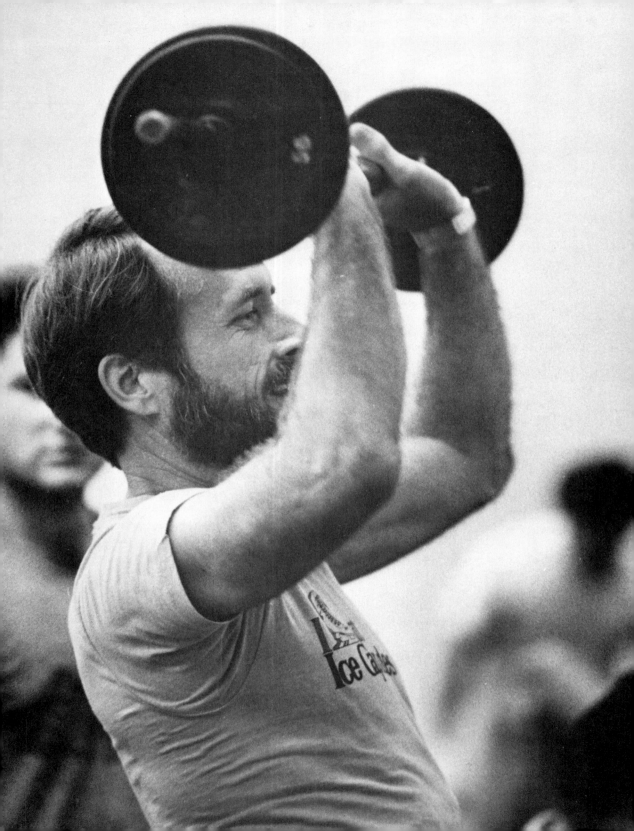

5

Putting Your Program Together

Now that you know how to do a variety of exercises, putting your strength training program together is easy if you incorporate the principles and concepts outlined in Chapter 2. You'll remember that one basic characteristic of your quality program must be periodic repetition and another must be compatibility with your goals and abilities. Since many of you may be new to or have limited experience with strength training, we'll start by discussing several simple three-day-a-week programs. Later we'll go over examples of more complex and advanced programs. Remember: *You should try to use as uncomplicated a program as possible, so long as it gives you favorable results.* Never start with an advanced, sophisticated program. If you do, then when progress drops off you'll find it difficult to change the program in such a way as to restimulate progress. Advanced training techniques are like tools. If you use them all initially, what will you have left to use when they wear out?

When beginning your program, work slowly, with light weights, and keep the program simple.

TWO SIMPLE GROUPS OF EXERCISES

A three-training-day-a-week program has been found by experiment and practical experience to produce excellent results even for reasonably experienced trainees. It satisfies the periodic repetition principle, and, if weight training is your primary means of exercise, it satisfies the generally accepted concept that three workouts a week of about one hour each is the minimum amount of exercise compatible with good health.

We know that the first principle of a quality program is to include a period of warm-up, preferably with stretching, at the start of each workout.

The next step in constructing your program is to pick exercises from those you learned in the last chapter, being sure to satisfy the principle of completeness and simplicity. As reasonable suggestions, consider the two groups of exercises listed below:

Set A	Purpose	Set B
1. Bench press	Upper-body pushing	1. Incline press
2. Leg press	Leg and hip extension	2. Lunge
3. Upright row	Upper-body pulling	3. Shoulder shrug
4. Machine leg curl	Hamstring work	4. Boot leg curl
5. Pull-up	Upper-body pulling	5. Lat pull-down
6. Good morning	Low back work	6. Stiff leg deadlift
7. Trunk curl	Abdominal work	7. Leg raise

Note that both groups satisfy the "complete and simple" principle. A fast and easy way to check this important point is to ask yourself if an upper-body pushing and pulling movement and a leg and hip thrusting (extension) movement have been included with torso strengthening exercises. In both Set A and Set B, exercises 6 and 7 are for torso strengthening (abdominals and lower back), exercises 3 and 5 are upper-body pulling exercises, exercise 1 is an upper-body pushing exercise, and exercise 2 is a leg and hip thrusting movement. You probably should review these classifications in Chapter 4. Doing exercise 4 in either set helps balance strength development for knee flexion (hamstring muscles) with the knee extension strength developed by exercise 2. Thus, you could replace any exercise in Set A with the same numbered exercise from Set B without affecting the completeness of the program. Or, a number of other exercises from Chapter 4 could be substituted, for example, an upper-body pulling movement, such as the dumbbell row. Also, a second upper-body pushing movement, such as the overhead press, could be added to the exercises of either Set A or Set B to place more emphasis on your pecs, triceps, or anterior deltoids.

The point is, you can use many different collections of exercises to form a reasonable program, just so long as you satisfy the "complete and simple" principle, and don't overdo it. Maybe one upper-body pulling exercise is enough for you to start with, rather than two as given in Sets A and B above. The program must be compatible with your abilities, and it's better to do too little work with a muscle group than too much. Later on, I'll show you example programs with as few as five, and as many as 12, exercises in them.

OTHER POINTS TO CONSIDER

So far we have taken a number of steps in constructing the first basic example program. We know you'll train three days every week (Monday-Wednesday-Friday, Monday-Thursday-Saturday, etc.), that you'll do warm-up exercises at the start of each workout (discussed in detail in Chapter 2), and that the program will consist of seven exercises (Set A or Set B). But we're not finished yet. We still have to decide whether you will use a priority or a circuit system, how many sets and reps of each exercise you will do, and how much weight you will use for each exercise in your workouts. These decisions depend largely on your goals.

Circuit or Priority System?

If muscular endurance and cardiovascular fitness are your primary goals, then a circuit system will probably be most efficient to achieve them. You should do the circuit with little or no rest between stations (or do light aerobic exercise between stations), with higher reps per set (10 to 15), and a greater number of excursions through the circuit—perhaps 5 to 10. As mentioned in Chapter 2, you'll find that this program design will force you to use less weight in each exercise, relative to your maximum, than would be possible with most other program designs, since you're constantly on the move with little or no rest. The weight you use in each exercise should permit you to do the scheduled number of reps—let's say 15—but the last one or two should be difficult to complete, especially the final time or two through the circuit. This is particularly true on the training days that you plan to be heavy ones. (More on light, medium, and heavy training days shortly.)

If your training goal is primarily strength development, you could still use a circuit system, but with the modifications discussed at the end of Chapter 3, namely, rest between stations, lower reps per set, and heavier weights relative to your maximum. A *priority system* however, is the most productive. *When you're going for strength gains,* with a priority system you would do, say, the exercises in Set A, in the order of their importance to you relative to your goals.

A general rule is to do the exercises that involve the largest muscle groups first. Thus, if leg and hip strength development is most important to you, do all sets of leg presses first. If upper-body strength is most important to you, do bench presses first. Put the rest of the exercises in an order so that smaller muscle groups or single-joint movement exercises, such as leg curls, which involve only knee flexion, come last.

Let's say that upper-body strength is your priority; a reasonable order for Set A in a priority system would be:

1. Bench press (many muscles of the upper body involved)
2. Leg press (large leg and hip extensors)
3. Good morning (large back and hip extensors)
4. Pull-up (large upper back muscles)
5. Trunk curl (abdominals)
6. Upright row (shoulder and shoulder girdle muscles)
7. Leg curl (hamstrings)

Trunk curls were placed between the pull-up and upright row because the latter two both involve the arms and shoulders. Placing them back to back would not give the elbow flexor muscles rest time, and would force you to use less weight in the upright row. *Remember, if strength is your goal, you should use as much weight as possible on heavy training days for the number of repetitions you're scheduled to do.* Keep in mind as you set up your priorities that the exact exercises used always influence the order to some extent, despite the general guidelines given above. For example, if you decide to do lunges or squats rather than leg presses, then good mornings should not follow, since the back muscles (spinal erectors) are worked heavily in both exercises. Instead, place an exercise not involving the back muscles in between.

How Many Sets and Reps?

Once you've determined the order of exercises in your priority system, you must decide how many sets and reps to do. Since we are now considering strength as a primary goal, you will want to handle fairly heavy weights relative to your maximum in each movement. Classic studies by the strength training pioneers Drs. Richard Berger and John "Pat" O'Shea in the early and mid-1960s indicated that three sets of five or six reps in core exercises (that is, those, such as bench presses or squats, that work larger muscle groups), performed three days a week, resulted in greater strength gains than do other set and rep combinations. Because of these research results, many people do three sets of five or six reps in the major exercises in their program. This is a productive way to train, and doing three sets of five reps in the bench press, then in the leg press, and so on, as listed above will certainly result in good strength gains. I recommend, though, that you do more reps than this in abdominal work and other exercises that work smaller muscles or single muscle groups. In leg curls, for example, do 10 to 15 reps.

Limitations

There are, however, some other considerations. The studies done by Berger and O'Shea typically involved college-aged students participating in a required weight training class. The experiments with these classes continued anywhere from 6 to 12 weeks. People respond to a given weight training program differently depending on previous strength training experience, exercise background in general, age, and genetic traits. There is no assurance, for example, that a middle-aged person who has already trained regularly with weights for a 10-year period would make the best strength gains by doing three sets of five reps in core exercises, as the novice college students did. Also, and perhaps most important, what happens to progress after 6, 10, or 12 weeks of three sets of five reps? Can progress be maintained? This is where the ideas about variation of training programs and training cycles become critical.

Before getting into details with additional examples, let's try to develop an understanding of why these variational methods work by discussing a generalized theory about the stages and processes your body goes through while trying to adapt to regular exercise.

THE GENERAL ADAPTATION SYNDROME

A theory formulated in the middle of this century by Dr. Hans Selye is sometimes called his "stress theory," but more commonly the General Adaptation Syndrome. "GAS" provides a framework from which most exercise programs and training cycles can be designed. Dr. Selye's clinical observations with humans and experiments with mice and rats led him to propose a three-stage process employed by any living organism when adapting to a stimulus that tends to disrupt its normal functional state *(homeostasis)*. The disrupting stimulus is called a *stressor* and may be beneficial (exercise) or harmful (germs). GAS proposes that when any stressor—such as physical trauma, infection, heat, fright—is imposed on a living organism, the organism's initial response results in a decrease in its ability to cope with additional stressors. This is called the *shock* or *initial alarm stage* of GAS. If you are exposed to a flu virus, for example, your ability to cope with exercise is greatly reduced. As time passes after the stressor exposure, however, your body should make internal adjustments that result in adaptations so that future exposure to the original stressor in particular, and to other stressors in general, will be less disrupting to homeostasis.

Reversal of the shock phase is termed *counter shock,* and it leads to the *resistance phase* of GAS. The effect of adaptation to a given stressor on your body's ability to cope with other stressors is called *cross-resistance.* This is why, for example, a person who stays in shape through regular exercise can better withstand the pressures of work or the common cold.

If multiple stressors are imposed on your body, counter shock may not occur, or the resistance phase may deteriorate into the third or exhaustion phase of GAS. The possible negative effects of multiple stressors is referred to as *cross-sensitization.* Failure to recover from the shock phase, or the exhaustion phase of GAS, may also occur from a single very potent stressor, or exposure to a given stressor for a prolonged period of time. Severe physical trauma from a car crash, for example, may result in death. In a less extreme illustration, heavy physical exercise day after day for many weeks will probably result in "overtraining," which is a manifestation of the *exhaustion phase* of GAS.

The phasic structure of Dr. Seyle's adaptation theory is the basis for the concept of variation and training cycles for both general exercise and specialized conditioning for athletes at all competitive levels—as we shall see in this chapter and in Chapter 7.'

An additional and very important concept of GAS is that of the body's *specific* and *non-specific* responses to stressors. The adaptations we discussed in Chapter 2 for muscle fibers were, of course, specific to the exercise demands made on the fibers (exercise specificity principle). The new concept here is that *no matter* what type of exercise demand, or what stressor in general, is imposed on your body, *a non-specific response will also occur.* Non-specific responses affect your body as a whole through the nervous system and hormonal and other biochemical processes.

The ultimate concept for you to grasp is that *all stressors* of whatever type *result in essentially the same non-specific effects in addition to their own specific effects.* A burned finger elicits a specific response to guard against infection and

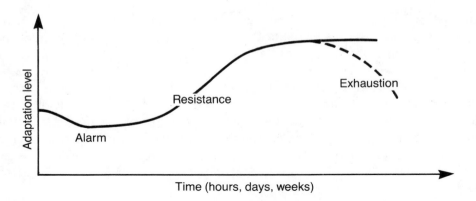

Graphical representation of the three phases of the general adaptation syndrome

repair damaged tissue, plus a non-specific response. A strenuous workout program results in specific bodily adaptations and the *same* non-specific responses that were caused by the burned finger, or the pressure at work, or the term paper due next week. Since non-specific stressor responses are additive, the exhaustion phase of GAS may result as a cumulative effect of many seemingly minor stressors.

Thus, in planning your exercise program, it is prudent to consider the other stressors in your daily life, as well as during special periods of abnormal pressure and commitments. World-class athletes in a number of countries are monitored regularly for signs of excess stress, which is technically defined as the total result of bodily responses to stressors. Typically their blood and urine parameters are monitored, as well as their resting heart rate and blood pressure. You, however, can suspect excess stress if you experience a loss of appetite and weight, sleep disorders, gastrointestinal ulcers, a lack of, or decrement in, training progress, or just a general feeling of constant fatigue and ill health. The fastest and only real cure for this problem, if indeed it is a manifestation of the exhaustion phase of adaptation, is to decrease the level of stressors acting on your body. Maybe you need to take a vacation, or to reduce the intensity and duration of your exercise program, or to cut back on other activities—whatever you can manage at the time.

Application of GAS

An application of the above theory to exercise program planning indicates that (1) exercise programs should start gradually to ease through the shock or initial alarm phase of GAS, and then slowly, over a period of weeks, intensify to the desired level (an initial decrease in your strength or physical feeling may occur, this is the alarm stage of GAS); (2) the content, intensity, and duration of workouts should *not* remain constant, since the body could rapidly adapt to a constant stressor level and improvement would stop; and (3) occasional breaks or layoffs from your regular exercise program are needed to reduce and change stressor input to your body, and thus to avoid the exhaustion phase of GAS. Typical periods to apply these three concepts are one or two weeks for an initial phase of training (or so-called readaptation after a layoff), six to ten weeks for the major portion of a training cycle, and one or two weeks for a break or, better still, a change to some other physical activities resulting in what's referred to as "active rest."

GAS is cyclical and fluctuating in nature, and by training in a similar manner you can expect to make greater gains over longer periods.

The basic ideas of GAS can also be applied to responses of your body that occur over other periods. You can consider, for example, a single one- or two-hour workout as composed of a shock phase at the start when you feel tight and uncomfortable, followed by a resistance phase once you're "warmed-up" and accustomed to the activity level, and finally an exhaustion phase when fatigue sets in. Dr. Selye himself has made an analogy of GAS to the human lifespan by analyzing characteristics of childhood, adulthood, and old age. For the purposes of conditioning our bodies, training cycles of a few months' duration will be the main focus of examples applying GAS to exercise in this chapter and Chapter 7. After a few examples that illustrate additional important concepts, I'll show you a specific strength training cycle.

HEAVY, LIGHT, AND MEDIUM WORKOUTS—HOW TO QUANTIFY THEM

At the beginning of this chapter, we saw how to use the principles of completeness and simplicity to pick two appropriate groups of exercises for a strength training program. We then discussed how to use such a group of exercises in a circuit system to emphasize either muscular endurance and cardiovascular fitness (higher reps, etc.) or strength (lower reps, etc.). We also learned about a priority system workout and how to pick sets and reps to maximize strength gains. All those examples are productive programs that you can use according to your goals and lifting experience. But all programs have limitations. The following examples will illustrate techniques, programs, and cycles that will

permit you to effectively utilize the guidelines of GAS in a variety of ways.
Consider the following workout:*

1. *Power clean:* 80 × 5 (meaning 5 reps with 80 pounds), 100 × 5 × 3
(meaning three sets of five reps with 100 pounds)
      Total: 20 reps, 1,900 pounds
2. *Bench press:* 100 × 5, 120 × 5 × 3
      Total: 20 reps, 2,300 pounds
3. *Parallel squat:* 120 × 5, 140 × 5 × 3
      Total: 20 reps, 2,700 pounds

   Grand total: 60 reps, 6,900 pounds
4. *Leg curls:* 20 × 10, 30 × 10 × 2
5. *Sit-ups:* 2 sets of 25 reps

Volume: 60 reps
Load: 6,900 pounds
Intensity: $\dfrac{Load}{Volume} = \dfrac{6{,}900 \text{ pounds}}{60 \text{ reps}} = 115$ pounds per rep

There are a number of interesting features about this type of workout and the method used to evaluate it quantitatively (that is, describe it objectively by numbers). It is based on three core exercises and two assistance exercises. Yet with only five total exercises (simplicity), it satisfies the completeness characteristic of a quality program, working all the major muscle groups of the legs, hips, torso, back, chest, shoulders, and arms. Quantitatively, the volume for each exercise is the total number of lifts done in that exercise—20 in the above example; and the volume of the workout as a whole is the total number of lifts (repetitions) done during the entire workout—60 in the above example. Reps should be counted only for major exercises, so leg curls and sit-ups are not included in the above example calculation. Additional examples that follow will help you decide which exercises to include in volume counts for your workouts. The volume in major lifting movements is important to consider, since it represents a quick estimate of the total effort demanded from your body during a workout.

Load is an even more accurate calculation of the work your body does.

---

*This example and the two that follow are an expansion of ideas presented in Bill Starr's book *The Strongest Shall Survive—Strength Training for Football,* listed under "Further Readings" at the end of the book.

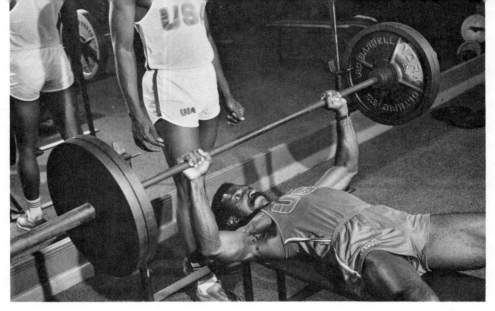

Training volume equals the total number of lifts per workout and should only be counted for the major exercises, such as the bench press.

A load measurement is obtained simply by multiplying the weight used in each set by the number of reps, and adding the values from the whole workout together. In the bench press of the example above, 100 × 5 = 500, plus 120 × 5 × 3 = 1,800, for a load of 2,300 pounds. The same is then done for the other core exercises. By themselves, load figures would not be of much more value than volume figures in quantifying the total demands or stressors imposed on your body by a given workout. By dividing the load figure by the volume figure, however, you get the very important and useful parameter of *intensity*.

Volume and intensity considered together clearly define the effort required by a given workout. Think of it this way: *Volume* is a measure of *quantity of work,* just as the distance covered by a jogger during a run, or the number of jumps or throws by a track-and-field athlete in a workout is a quantity measure. *Intensity,* on the other hand, is a measure of *quality of exercise.* For a jogger, intensity would correspond to his running speed and is measured in average minutes per mile—for example, 8.5 minutes per mile. For throwers and jumpers, intensity is the average distance thrown or jumped during the workout. In weight training, *intensity* is simply the average weight lifted per repetition. As seen in the example, it is calculated as total weight lifted (load) divided by total repetitions (volume). In other words, *intensity equals load over volume (I = L/V).*

In our example above, the heaviest weight lifted was 140 pounds, in the squat. The lightest weight lifted in a major exercise was 80 pounds, during warm-up for power cleans. By calculating load and volume as shown, the intensity formula $(I = L/V)$ tells us that the average weight lifted was 115 pounds per rep.

The absolute value of volume and intensity for your training sessions is important in analyzing workouts, planning future workouts, and measuring improvement. For example, I have mentioned the concept of having heavy, light, and medium training days in your strength program. Let's assume the workout just analyzed was your heavy day. The next workout should be light, which means about 75 to 85 percent as hard as the heavy day. We'll use approximately 80 percent of the heavy-day weights as an example.*

Light day (about 80 percent of previous heavy day)

1. *Power clean:* 65 × 5, 80 × 5 × 3
   Total: 20 reps, 1,525 pounds
2. *Bench press:* 80 × 5, 95 × 5 × 3
   Total: 20 reps, 1,825 pounds
3. *Parallel squat:* 95 × 5, 110 × 5 × 3
   Total: 20 reps, 2,125 pounds

   Grand total: 60 reps, 5,475 pounds
4. *Leg curls:* 20 × 10 × 3
5. *Sit-ups:* two sets of 25 reps

   Volume: 60 reps
   Load: 5,475 pounds
   Intensity: $5,475/60 = 91$ pounds per rep

The third workout of your training week should be medium in the demands it places on your body, and be in the range of about 85 to 95 percent of the heavy day. We'll use approximately 90 percent of the heavy-day weights for our example.

---

*Either before or after studying the next two examples, which also calculate V, L, and I, you may want to test your ability to determine these values from the weights, sets, and reps listed in the following sample workout:

1. *Power clean:* 50 × 5, 60 × 4, 70 × 3, 80 × 2, 85 × 1, 50 × 3
2. *Bench press:* 40 × 8, 50 × 6, 60 × 4, 75 × 2, 85 × 1, 50 × 5
3. *Parallel squat:* 75 × 5, 90 × 5, 90 × 5, 90 × 5, 75 × 5

(*Answers:* $V = 69$ reps, $L = 4540$ pounds, $I = 65.8$ pounds per rep.)

Medium day (about 90 percent of the heavy-day weights)

1. *Power clean:* 70 × 5, 90 × 5 × 3
   Total: 20 reps, 1,700 pounds
2. *Bench press:* 90 × 5, 110 × 5 × 3
   Total: 20 reps, 2,100 pounds
3. *Parallel squats:* 110 × 5, 125 × 5 × 3
   Total: 20 reps, 2,425 pounds

   Grand total: 60 reps, 6,225 pounds
4. *Leg curls:* 20 × 10, 25 × 10 × 2
5. *Sit-ups:* 2 sets of 25 reps

   Volume: 60 reps
   Load: 6,225 pounds
   Intensity: 6,225/60 = 104 pounds per rep

The arithmetic for quantitative evaluation of the heavy, light, and medium workouts above shows that:

1. From workout to workout during a week, the training load and intensity have considerable variation—about 21 percent from the heavy (L = 6,900 pounds, I = 115 pounds per rep) to light (L = 5,475 pounds, I = 91 pounds per rep) day.

2. The absolute volume, or total number of reps performed in core exercises, is constant from workout to workout (60) and, therefore, from week to week (180).

3. The total weekly load (6,900 + 5,475 + 6,225 pounds, or 18,600 pounds in all) will change little from week to week due to the relatively small changes possible week to week in exercise weights.

Point (1) is a favorable property of the program, although the variation from heavy to light day in load and intensity could be larger (30 percent to 40 percent) in more advanced programs. Point (2) is not a favorable property of the program but is acceptable and productive for beginners and for advanced trainees over shorter periods (two to four weeks). Programs for advanced trainees are generally designed to vary the volume, as well as the load and intensity, from workout to workout during a week. Likewise, total weekly volume can be adjusted occasionally as a means of introducing additional variation into a program. Making these types of adjustments helps avoid the unfavorable property of the current example listed as point (3) above.

Volume, load, and intensity were introduced with this example because the calculations and meaning of the values should be easier for you to follow here than with a more complex example. The examples that follow will illustrate additional ways to plan strength programs, and the methods of quantitative analysis just introduced will be used to pick out the good and bad features of each program.

WHEN AND HOW MUCH TO INCREASE WEIGHTS

Before going on to new examples, I should point out that if you actually use the current example program, or any program using H-L-M days (which means almost all programs!), the weights are increased on a heavy day if you completed all sets and reps successfully on the heavy day of the previous week. In the current example, power cleans may increase to $105 \times 5 \times 3$, bench presses to $125 \times 5 \times 3$, and squats to $150 \times 5 \times 3$. These represent increases of about 5 percent, which are very manageable for a beginner. In your first weeks of strength training you may be able to increase a little more than this, but don't push yourself too hard. More advanced lifters may make increases of only 2 or 3 percent, such as from 200 pounds to 205 pounds, in a given exercise. Warm-up sets can also be increased slightly. With the above changes, the intensity of the heavy-day workout would increase from 115 to about 122 pounds per rep (see if you can do the calculations to get $I = 122$). Since light and medium days are percentages of the heavy day, the weights handled on these days and the resulting intensity would also increase. This type of program should be followed for about 10 weeks, after which some type of change is needed, as indicated by the guidelines based on GAS. A number of changes are possible, such as different exercises, more or fewer sets and reps, or a whole new program design—perhaps four workouts a week rather than three. Some suggestions are presented in the following examples.

THE SINGLE-HEAVY-EXERCISE-PER-DAY PROGRAM— ITS LIMITATIONS

You may find it difficult, both physically and psychologically, to push yourself to a limit in three or more core exercises on the same (heavy) day. One seeming solution to this potential problem that some people try is to go heavy in only one exercise each day. Here's a sample program, modified from the previous example, but using the same set, rep, and weight values for each exercise on different days. You may find this type of program attractive, but be warned: It does have certain limitations, as we'll see.

Monday

1. *Power clean* (heavy—20 reps, 1,900 pounds)
2. *Bench press* (medium—20 reps, 2,100 pounds)
3. *Full squat* (light—20 reps, 2,125 pounds)
4. *Secondary exercises* (leg curls, sit-ups)
   Total: 60 reps, 6,125 pounds
   Volume: 60 reps
   Load: 6,125 pounds
   Intensity: 6,125/60 = 102 pounds

Wednesday

1. *Bench press* (heavy—20 reps, 2,300 pounds)
2. *Full squat* (medium—20 reps, 2,425 pounds)
3. *Power clean* (light—20 reps, 1,525 pounds)
4. *Secondary exercises* (leg curls, sit-ups)
   Total: 60 reps, 6,250 pounds
   Volume: 60 reps
   Load: 6,250 pounds
   Intensity: 6,250/60 = 104 pounds

Friday

1. *Full squat* (heavy—20 reps, 2,700 pounds)
2. *Power clean* (medium—20 reps, 1,700 pounds)
3. *Bench press* (light—20 reps, 1,825 pounds)
4. *Secondary exercises* (leg curls, sit-ups)
   Total: 60 reps, 6,225 pounds
   Volume: 60 reps
   Load: 6,225 pounds
   Intensity: 6,225/60 = 104 pounds

Note that in this system, on each day you first do the exercise in which you are going heavy, then the medium, and then the light exercise. (Again, the values for volume and load are taken from H, L, or M days of the previous example.) The exercise done heavy on one day is done light on the following training day. Thus, you need to do only one exercise heavy each day! That may sound great, but there are problems with this type of program design, which are easily seen by looking at the volume, load, and intensity numbers. The absolute volume is 60 reps per day because of the program structure, as was the case with the previous example. But the load and intensity values give us very important information: namely, *there is very little variation in this program.* The daily load ranges from 6,125 to 6,250 pounds, and the intensity from 102 to 104 pounds per rep. Compare these values with those in the standard H-L-M program first presented, where the load ranged from 5,475 to 6,900 pounds, and the intensity from 91 to 115 pounds per rep. That's quite a difference, and there are two significant points to consider:

1. As you develop a larger and larger backlog of strength training, the variation of load and intensity in the weekly training cycle becomes critical. A beginner (roughly the first year) can generally make good progress with little or no variation. With more training experience, however, variation becomes necessary, based on the ideas of GAS, and even that shown earlier in the standard H-L-M program could be insufficient.

2. Remember that strength training may be only one part of your total conditioning program. Programs similar to the earlier example of a standard H-L-M program might fit in very well with other training. On the light day, more time could be spent on the court or field or in the water. The heavy day might be the only one that requires a considerable cutback in other training or physical activity. By contrast, the "single heavy exercise per day" type of program might not fit in so well with your other physical activities, since every day is about the same in load and intensity. Other activities might reduce the weight you can handle in the heavy exercise, reducing the strength training stimulus, or, if you lift weights first, muscle fatigue may decrease your performance in or enjoyment of the physical activities you do next.

Thus, the "single heavy exercise per day" type of program just presented has definite limitations. It can be productive if you're a beginner or if you're a more advanced trainee and use it for a few weeks as a change from the standard H-L-M system to handle heavier weights in each of the core exercises (since you wouldn't be doing heavy lifts in each on the same day, you won't be as fatigued).

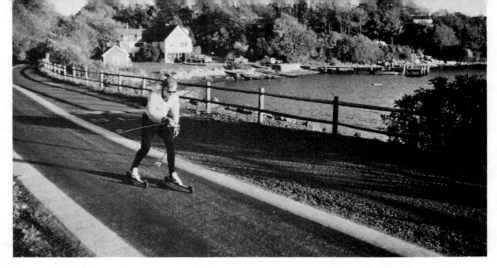

The single-heavy-exercise-per-workout approach combines well with other training such as roller-ski workouts for cross-country skiing.

EXERCISE SUBSTITUTION AND SET-REP VARIATION

There are ways to add additional variation to either the standard H-L-M or the "single heavy exercise per day" type of program. If you simply change the core exercises occasionally—perhaps the power clean to a deadlift and shrug, bench press to an incline press, and squat to a lunge—you do add variation though the unfavorable characteristic of constant daily and weekly volume will remain. *If, however, you use one substitute exercise each day, as shown below, and also change the number of sets and reps for that exercise from what would have been used for the original exercise, then the daily volume can be made to fluctuate.* With intelligent planning, this procedure will add variation to your daily volume while maintaining it for load and intensity.

As an illustration of adding variety to your weekly exercise movements and daily volume, let's *use a substitute exercise to replace a core exercise on either its light or its medium day in the previous "single heavy exercise per day" program.* The substitute exercise should work the same muscle groups, in a similar movement pattern, as the original core exercise. It should usually be a movement in which you can handle less weight than in the original exercise. Otherwise, the light or medium nature (on that workout day) of the exercise that it's replacing will be lost.

In the following example, notice the substitutions made in the previous "single heavy exercise per day" program listed on page 160 (they are marked with an asterisk *), and the set and rep (volume) changes.

1. Power clean (heavy)—4 sets of 5 reps ($V = 20$)
2. Bench press (medium)—4 sets of 5 reps ($V = 20$)
3. *Front squat or leg press—3 sets of 10 reps ($V = 30$)
4. Secondary exercises
   Total volume: $20 + 20 + 30 = 70$ reps

Wednesday

1. Bench press (heavy)—4 sets of 5 reps ($V = 20$)
2. Full squat (medium)—4 sets of 5 reps ($V = 20$)
3. *Snatch or clean from knee level—3 sets of 3 reps ($V = 9$)
4. Secondary exercises
   Total volume: $20 + 20 + 9 = 49$ reps

Friday

1. Full squat (heavy)—4 sets of 5 reps ($V = 20$)
2. Power clean (medium)—4 sets of 5 reps ($V = 20$)
3. *Incline press or overhead press—4 sets of 5 reps ($V = 20$)
4. Secondary exercises
   Total volume: $20 + 20 + 20 = 60$ reps

In this example, the substitutions were made for core exercises on the day they were to have been done lightly. The substitutions could have been made on one or more medium days instead, or occasionally a heavy day could be used to go to your maximum in the replacement exercise. The reason for doing 3 × 10, 3 × 3, and 4 × 5 in the substitute exercises is that they are productive set-rep combinations that will vary the daily volume.

Even the original core exercise set-rep combinations could be changed to achieve the desired daily volume changes. Doing 3 × 5 (= 15 reps) rather than 4 × 5 (= 20 reps) could be used on a light day for a given core exercise to reduce that day's volume.

The possibilities for variation are many, so you must use your common sense, background knowledge, and experience to make proper choices based on your goals and capabilities. Three to six sets is a common range, as is 3 to 10 or 15 reps. But remember things like the physiological differences in doing low versus high reps (Chapter 2), and the effects of different rest intervals between sets, when planning the details of your strength and overall conditioning program.

Before moving on, you should be aware of a few other important points:

1. All the example programs given so far could be done in either a circuit or a priority system.

2. The past three examples used quantitative calculations that involved only the core exercises, but the total programs should include several secondary exercises, such as abdominal work and leg curls. These do not have to be done as hard as the core movements—that is, they needn't require as many sets, or as high a percentage of maximum weight—and do not need as much variation unless they serve an unusually important purpose in the program.

3. Keep a written record of all your workouts so that you can analyze and accurately monitor your progress. Believe me, you will forget workout details if you don't record them. Also write down outside influences that may affect you, such as lack of sleep, exams at school, or overtime at work. With an inexpensive pocket calculator, you can easily do the arithmetic to determine the volume, load, and intensity of your workouts from the data in your notebook.

HOW TO CHANGE VOLUME WEEK TO WEEK—THE UNLOAD WEEK METHOD

Up to this point, we've paid little attention to total *weekly* (as opposed to daily) volume, load, and intensity changes, other than noting that they changed little, if at all, from week to week in our example programs. There are several methods to vary weekly volume, load, and intensity, just as there are to vary them daily.

Perhaps the simplest and most effective is called *the unload week method,* which is often used by competitive lifters. It works like this: After every two or three weeks of hard training, depending on your experience level and the duration of your current program, you plan an overall light week. The light week has considerably lower total volume and load, and lower intensity. Let's say, for example, you're doing core exercises for four sets of five reps during the heavier "work" weeks. During the unload week you could do them for three sets of three reps. For three core exercises, the total weekly volume would drop from 180 reps in the work weeks (4 sets $\times$ 5 reps $\times$ 3 exercises $\times$ 3 days) to 81 reps (3 $\times$ 3 $\times$ 3 $\times$ 3) in the unload week (a 44 percent decrease!). This is more of a reduction than needed to produce sufficient variation, but it is typical of what some top competitors actually do. Normal ranges for unload-week decreases are five or six sets dropping to three, ten reps per set dropping to five or six, and five or six reps per set dropping to three. The total weekly volume decrease should be in the range of 30 to 50 percent. The amount of weight used in each exercise drops much less, maybe 10 percent each day of the week, resulting in about a 10 percent reduction in intensity for the unload week. As an example, let's look at what happens with one core exercise, such as the overhead press. During a work week on the heavy day, you might be doing $80 \times 5 \times 3$ so that $V = 15$, $L = 1,200$, $I = 80$. A good choice for the unload week would be $70 \times 3 \times 3$ so that $V = 9$, $L = 630$, $I = 70$. V was reduced 40 percent; L, 47 percent; and I, 12 percent.

Remember, this is only one method for varying weekly volume, load, and intensity. Others involve adding or excluding assistance, and even core exercises, from week to week, or changing the number of training days per week to produce the desired program variation. These methods are *all* advanced, and you needn't worry about unload weeks until you've been training for at least a few months, and maybe a year or more, depending on your physical condition and how your body responds to exercise. GAS affects us all a little differently.

SPLIT-ROUTINE PROGRAMS

Some advanced trainees prefer to include a rather large number of exercises in their programs, perhaps more than a dozen. Limitations on time and energy for one workout make it necessary to divide the exercises used into two groups performed on alternate days. This training format is called a "split-routine" program. Bodybuilders generally use this type of system. They may use one group of exercises involving primarily arm, chest, and abdominal muscles and a second group working back, leg, and hip muscles. A split routine can work well even for beginners, if fewer total exercises are used. It is particularly helpful if limited time is available for each workout—your lunch hour, for example—but you can train four to six days a week.

Here are typical sample groupings for a split-routine program that could work well for many of you.

Group 1	Group 2
Bench press	Lunges
Dumbbell flys	Shoulder shrugs
Overhead press	Leg curls
Dumbbell curls	Lat pull-downs
Tricep press	Stiff leg deadlift
Trunk curls	Calf raises

Group 1 exercises could be done Monday and Thursday with Group 2 exercises done Tuesday and Friday, resulting in a four-workout-a-week program. This schedule allows one workout a week to be a heavy day for each group, with the other days light to medium. If you are an advanced trainee, you can intensify the program by doing *each* group three days a week, following the heavy-light-medium system. A possible scheme for one week of training would look like this:

Day	M	Tu	W	Th	F	Sa	Su
Group 1	H	—	L	—	M	—	—
Group 2	—	M	—	H	—	L	—

Obviously, there can be other variations. In a split-routine program, the numbers of sets and reps are based on the considerations we've discussed previously. It is very common for bodybuilders to do 8 to 10 reps in most of the exercises in this type of program, since they want to do more work to burn more calories and keep their body fat low while they build up (hypertrophy) or define their muscles. Abdominal and calf exercises are usually done for higher reps—perhaps 20 or more, depending on the resistance. Load, volume, and intensity are calculated as shown in the previous examples. Trunk curls and calf raises are not generally counted due to the light weight, if any, typically used in the former, and the disproportionately high number of reps, short movement range, and heavy weights typical of the latter. But leg curls should be counted in this type of program if the weight used is comparable to that used in most of the other exercises in the program.

Since split-routine programs often involve dumbbell work, you should know how to calculate load, volume, and intensity for dumbbell exercises. If

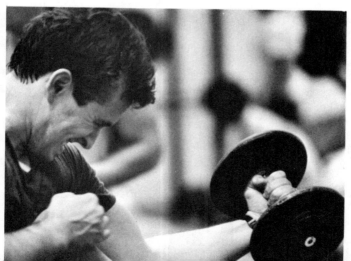

A split-routine program often involves dumbbell work.

you use dumbbells *simultaneously in each hand,* add their weight together and count the number of reps done. For example, dumbbell flys done for three sets of ten reps, with 20-pound dumbbells, would count as a volume of 30 reps and a load of 1,200 pounds (40 × 10 × 3). In this case $I = 1,200/30 = 40$ pounds, or twice the individual dumbbell's weight. If you use one dumbbell, first with one hand and then the other, use the weight of the dumbbell and add the number of reps done by each hand. For example, dumbbell rows done for three sets of eight reps with each hand, using a 30-pound dumbbell, would count as a volume of 48 reps and load of 1,440 pounds (30 × 16 × 3). Here $I = 1,440/48 = 30$ pounds, the weight of the single dumbbell used.*

"SUPER SETS"

The exercises in the sample split-routine program above could be done in a circuit each day (with some changes in order), but would more commonly be done in a priority system. Also, there's a technique called "super setting" that can be used in a priority system but should not involve "total body" exercises. It requires doing two related exercises consecutively, with no break. For example, if you did a set of dumbbell curls and followed it immediately (without rest) with a set of tricep presses, you'd have done a "super set" for the arm muscles. After a few minutes rest, this super set would be repeated. Typically, you'd do three super sets for each body part to be worked in this manner.

A super set usually works antagonistic muscle groups in a given area of the body, such as the upper arm in the example just given. This technique usually results in a "pumped up" feeling in the muscles used as they are being flushed with blood. This pumped or tight feeling is readily obtained when exercising smaller muscle groups, such as in the forearm, upper arm, and calf.

I *strongly discourage* anyone with cardiac problems from pumping their muscles up this way, since blood pressure rises to force blood through the tight muscles. If you fall into this category but have your doctor's OK to lift weights, emphasize exercises that work the larger muscle groups, or multiple muscle groups together, and never do super sets.

---

*As a test for yourself, calculate *V, L,* and *I* for the following workout:

1. *Incline dumbbell presses:* two 25-pound dumbbells for three sets of 10 reps
2. *Dumbbell rows:* a 40-pound dumbbell for three sets of 10 reps with each arm
3. *Upright rows:* a 50-pound barbell for three sets of eight reps

(*Answers:* $V = 114$ reps, $L = 5,100$ pounds, $I = 44.7$ pounds per rep.)

THE "CYCLIC" METHOD OF STRENGTH TRAINING

After you've trained with a fixed program or two over several months' time, or if you've been weight training in the past, the use of training cycle concepts could really help you increase or renew progress. A large amount of experimental evidence in this area has resulted from recent studies by Drs. Michael Stone and Harold O'Bryant. The basic plan of their research to compare cyclic strength training to a common conventional strength program is summarized by the accompanying table.

STRENGTH TRAINING CYCLE VERSUS CONVENTIONAL PROGRAM

Week:	1	2	3	4	5	6	7	8	9	10
Cycle group	3 sets of 10 reps			3 sets of 5 reps				3 sets of 3 reps		
Conventional	←			— 3 sets of 6 reps —						→

The same collection of exercises, mainly core movements such as bench presses and squats, was done by each group of subjects. As you can see, the conventional group subjects did 18 reps per day in each exercise (not counting warm-up lifts), while the cycle group did 30 reps per exercise per day during Weeks 1 through 3; 15 reps during Weeks 4 through 7, and 9 reps during Weeks 8 through 10. Thus, the cycle group had large variations in volume during the program. Intensity increases were also large for the cycle group, since considerably heavier weights could be used as the reps decreased from 10 to 5 to 3. The conventional group had no volume variation during the 10 weeks—18 reps per exercise every day—and little intensity increase, since the weight they lifted for three sets of six reps could be increased only gradually.

The results of this representative comparison were very impressive. The cycle group experienced significantly greater increases in strength (as measured in the bench press and squat lifts) and power (as measured with vertical jumps) at the end of the training period.

Many different groups of subjects have been tested in recent years in similar experiments, and the results have always been essentially the same: The cycle group always shows the greater strength and power improvement.

Each phase of such a cycle does not have to be three or four weeks long, as in the example, but the length of each phase should be similar. Phases of two to six weeks would be reasonable. The high-rep phase of this type of cycle helps build muscle tissue, reduce body fat, and prepare the body for more intense

work. The medium- and low-rep phases develop strength and power in the
"potentiated" muscle.

This sample strength training cycle is a straightforward way of applying the basic concepts of variation and the General Adaptation Syndrome. Variation during any one week can be introduced by the simple heavy-light-medium day system or by the more complex alterations discussed previously in this chapter. Additional components of your overall conditioning program, such as running, swimming, or tennis, can easily be blended in.

ADDITIONAL SET-REP SEQUENCES

The Plateau System

Remember our discussion in Chapter 2 about the relationship between the number of reps done per set and the goals of a circuit program? Higher reps for endurance, lower reps for strength, and so forth? The same ideas hold true for choosing reps in a priority system of training. Several examples presented earlier in this chapter involved a *plateau system,* in which, after warm-up, the weight stayed constant—for example, 100 × 5, 120 × 5, 120 × 5, 120 × 5. In a plateau-priority system it is not uncommon for advanced trainees to do as many as five sets at the highest weight. Five reps were used in many of our examples to emphasize strength gains. You can use the same type of plateau system with higher or lower reps per set depending on your goals or the phase of a training cycle you are in.

The Step System

Another system of sets and reps is to keep the reps fixed—say, three per set—but increase the weight in each set until a maximum is reached. An example would be 80 × 3, 90 × 3, 100 × 3, 110 × 3, 120 × 3, 130 × 3. I don't highly recommend this system, but you can use it occasionally for variety, perhaps, in place of 80 × 3, 100 × 3, 120 × 3, 120 × 3, 120 × 3, or for determining the maximum weight you could lift for three reps of a given exercise. All the warm-up sets in the above sequence will tend to hold the maximum weight down a little, especially if you're doing more than three reps per set, but you can still get a good estimate of your 3RM—that is, maximum weight for three reps, or 3 Rep Max.

The Pyramid System

The pyramid system of sets and reps, too, can be used to add variety to your program. It also can be used to estimate your 1 RM—the maximum weight you can lift for one rep in an exercise. In a pyramid, the weight used in each set increases while the reps per set decrease. An example would be 80 × 10, 90 × 8, 100 × 6, 115 × 4, 130 × 2, 140 × 1, 100 × 5. Note that the last set calls for medium weight and reps for the purpose of "tapering off," rather than stopping abruptly, after a maximum weight.

Pyramids are generally used only with core-type exercises, not assistance or single-joint exercises. Pyramids can occasionally be used to add variety to a plateau system program, or can be used for a separate phase of a cycle. For example, three weeks of 12 rep sets, three weeks of 6 rep sets, three weeks of 3 rep sets, and three weeks of pyramids. This would probably be followed by a week off from weight training before starting a new cycle.

The Reverse-Pyramid System

Some people also "reverse" the pyramid. For example, they might do sets of 8, 6, 4, 2, 1, 2, 4, 6, 8 reps, with the weight increasing as the reps decrease and decreasing as the reps increase. This sequence represents a lot of work and I don't recommend it for most trainees. Also, I strongly advise against doing a *pure reverse pyramid,* such as 1, 2, 4, 6, 8, 10 reps, since such a sequence lacks specific warm-up. The idea behind a pure reverse pyramid is that it allows you to handle the heaviest weight before any fatigue develops. It is true that all the sets and reps before the single rep set in a standard pyramid will cause some fatigue and slightly decrease the maximum weight you can lift. But if you are in good shape, the effect will be small. If you want to lift a truer maximum, simply warm up with low rep sets—but always warm up before lifting heavy weights. A typical sequence, if your maximum squat were, for example, 120 pounds, would be 60 × 3, 80 × 3, 100 × 2, 115 × 1, 125 × 1 (for a new personal record, called a PR), 90 × 5.

MUSCULAR ENDURANCE AND ENDURANCE TRAINING

There are several important considerations relative to training for muscular endurance and endurance-oriented programs that you should keep in mind:

1. When muscle groups become stronger, they work at a lower percentage of their maximum contractile force when performing at a given absolute workload. This means they won't fatigue as fast at that workload as they would with the original strength level, which is an improvement in endurance. If you're a runner, for example, and initially have a maximum pace of 6 minutes per mile, then added leg and hip strength would result in that pace requiring a lower percentage of your maximal force output. This means you could run at that pace longer, or at a faster pace for the same length of time that you originally ran at the 6-minute-per-mile pace.

2. Using very high reps, 20 or more, is *not* the best way to develop muscular endurance for endurance-oriented activities. *It is better to use weight workouts to build strength and to rely on the endurance activity itself to build the endurance.* Increased strength, of course, will aid in developing endurance as discussed above. If, however, for some reason such as injury or bad weather, you can't do the endurance activity, then higher-rep sets in weight lifting can be a satisfactory short-term alternative.

3. Research has shown that endurance or aerobic-type exercise can have a negative effect on performance in explosive power-oriented activities, as well as on strength levels, particularly for highly trained strength-power athletes. Power refers to large forces being generated rapidly, as for sprinting, jumping, throwing, and Olympic-style weightlifting. Clearly, the fast-twitch-type muscle fibers, discussed in Chapter 1, with their high tension development and contraction speed, are important for power activities. Research into muscle adaptations has shown that with extensive aerobic exercise, fast twitch fibers can develop a large capability for oxidative metabolism, as with slow twitch fibers. This can be seen in the table of fiber adaptations on page 31. This type of fiber is then referred to as an "intermediate" fiber, with contraction tension and speed being between the typical values found for "normal" fast and slow twitch fibers. Such an adaptation is one important cause of the reduced power potential resulting from extensive endurance training.

You should not interpret the above information to mean that a strength-power athlete should never do any endurance type exercise. The recovery process after high intensity, short duration work is very dependent on oxidative metabolism. Thus, it is reasonable for even a power-oriented athlete to do some training that will maintain the oxidative system at an adequate level. Similarly, a long distance runner may need to sprint at the end of a race or retain a certain strength level in key muscle groups to maintain proper running form during a race. The value of an athlete including some of the apparently opposing types of exercise in training is real, but it must be done in proper amounts at selected times during a conditioning cycle. The concept of cycles in exercise programs can be important to you and everyone, not just athletes, and will be discussed again in Chapter 7.

SUMMARY

The sample programs presented in this chapter apply the principles we covered in earlier chapters. Some of the concepts illustrated in the examples are advanced, however, and you shouldn't try them if you're a beginner. To make good progress, neophytes need only choose exercises that satisfy the "completeness and simplicity" rule of Chapter 2, train with light, medium, and heavy workouts each week, and be progressive over a period of weeks, without missing workouts. As months and years go by, if you're a serious trainee, you will need to use more and more of the advanced training concepts presented to continue making progress. If you make the mistake of starting with very advanced training techniques, your initial progress is likely to be *no* faster than with a good basic program, and there will be little in the way of sophistication to add to improve your program as time goes by. In the long run, starting with advanced programs will shorten your years of progress.

Some individuals desire a strength and overall conditioning program that will get them "in shape." In the Introduction, I discussed the components of total physical fitness. Being in shape refers to a certain level of physical conditioning relative to muscular endurance, cardiovascular fitness, reasonable body fat levels, joint flexibility, and muscular strength and power. If you run the same distance at the same pace five days each week, or go through the same weight workout at the health spa three days each week, you will maintain a certain level of fitness. By the General Adaptation Syndrome, though, your level of fitness will not increase unless you increase the exercise stress level in a consistent way. Rather than being satisfied with a fixed fitness level, you can apply the concepts of variation presented in this chapter to your program and see real fitness improvement with little extra time or effort.

I should also mention that similar weight training programs can produce quite different results in similar individuals due to seemingly minor changes in factors such as reps per set and diet. Consider two similar individuals, A and B, who do the same five or six exercises three days each week. A does 10 or 12 reps per set and eats a balanced, low-calorie diet. B does five or six reps per set and eats everything in sight (the so-called "see food" diet). A would be

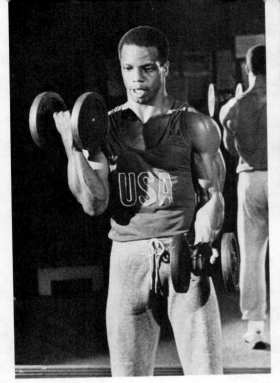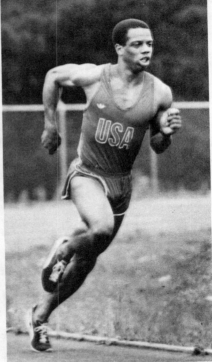

Your performance in certain "explosive" activities such as sprinting can be improved by doing appropriate weight movements fast.

expected to lose body fat, lose or maintain body weight, and develop stronger muscles with good definition. B would be expected to gain or maintain body fat, gain body weight, and develop larger and much stronger muscles but with less definition. Sex differences also affect the results of a given strength program. Women tend to develop less muscle size and definition and tend to maintain higher body fat levels, due to hormonal differences.

Finally, the speed at which you do the exercise movements also affects the way your body adapts to them. As a general rule, if the muscle groups being exercised are used "explosively" in the activity you are training for—such as Alpine skiing, sprinting in tennis, blocking in football, jumping in basketball or volleyball—then some of the time you should do appropriate exercise movements fast. This will help in neuromuscular learning—training your nervous system—and in the recruitment of fast motor units. It will also prepare your tendons and other connective tissues to better withstand rapidly developed forces and large accelerations. These considerations are obviously of great importance for athletes who in their sport are almost always moving in an explosive manner.

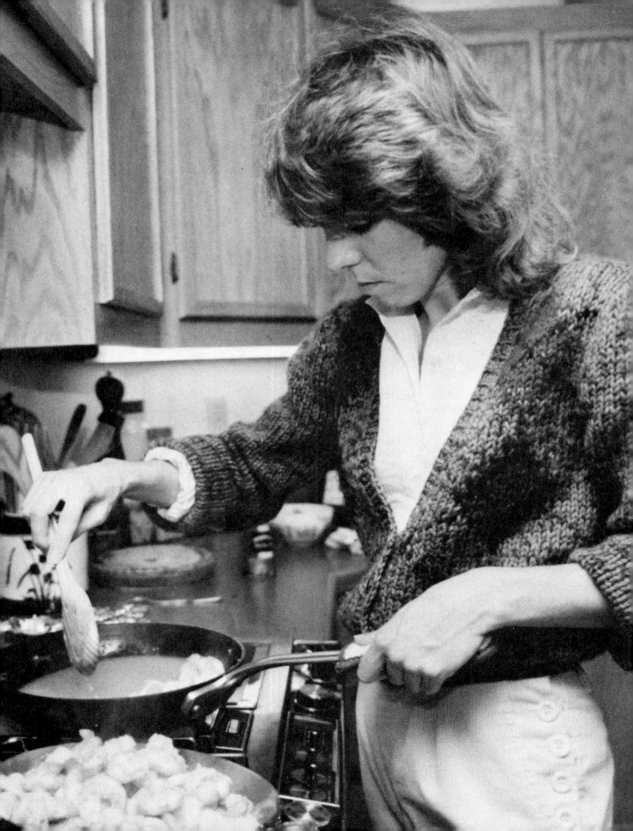

Nutrition

"A stomach full of food soothes by draining blood away from a disgruntled and maladapted brain."
—Dr. Hans Selye

The foods we eat should provide the quantity and variety of nutrients needed to meet the demands of our daily activities. This means that in addition to providing materials for building, repairing, and maintaining body tissues and structures, as well as regulating bodily processes, the foods we eat should meet our energy requirements. You are probably familiar with the different nutrient classifications: carbohydrates, proteins, fats, vitamins, minerals, and water. The first three supply all the bodily energy needs. Protein, fat, minerals, and water make up the various tissues and structures of the body. And vitamins, minerals, and water are important for proper regulation of bodily processes. Fiber is an additional substance found in many foods we eat. It is an indigestible (for humans) type of carbohydrate, such as cellulose, that aids in digestion and elimination.

Achieving a balanced diet is easy if you understand its components. For adults, it means consuming a good mix of foods from each of the four food groups. These include:

175

The food we eat should meet our daily energy requirements . . .

1. Meats, including fish, poultry and eggs
2. Dairy products, such as milk and cheese
3. Vegetables and fruits
4. Grain products, such as breads and cereals

Almost all basic books on nutrition discuss the food groups in some detail. Nutritionists generally recommend two to four servings daily from each group. Some substitutions are acceptable, such as cheese or nut mixtures rather than a meat serving.

When increasing or decreasing caloric intake, you should make proportionate adjustments in all food groups, by changing serving sizes or numbers, to keep the diet balanced.

CALORIC OR ENERGY BALANCE—WEIGHT GAIN OR LOSS

The energy content of foods is measured in terms of food calories. Each food calorie equals 1,000 "physical" calories. A physical calorie is the amount of heat energy needed to raise the temperature of one gram of water one degree Centigrade. Thus, one food calorie of energy will raise the temperature of 1,000 grams of water—which is the same as 1,000 milliliters or 1 liter of water—one degree Centigrade. For our purposes in this book *we'll use the single word "calorie" to mean food calorie.* If digestion and absorption factors are accounted for, the following energy content approximations, relative to food type, can be made:

1. One gram of carbohydrate = 4 calories
2. One gram of protein = 4 calories
3. One gram of fat = 9 calories

Since steady-state metabolism of foods requires oxygen to "burn" or metabolize the foods, the energy content may also be listed in terms of liters of oxygen consumed while foods are being used. There is some variation in energy yielded per unit of oxygen used to "burn" the three food types, but 5 calories per liter of oxygen is a reasonable approximation.

If you consistently consume more calories than you expend, a state of positive caloric balance exists, and excess calories are converted to, and primarily stored as, fat. If your caloric expenditure exceeds your caloric intake, a negative caloric balance exists and stored fat is metabolized.

Controlling and regulating caloric balance in humans involves complex processes. Genetics, culture, and habit play important roles. Short-term changes in caloric intake generally do not result in significant changes in body weight. Apparently, for most individuals there is a range of caloric intake and expenditure that must be exceeded consistently before body weight changes occur. Absorption and efficiency of utilization of food help explain the ability of some individuals to maintain body weight over long periods without trying, despite considerable fluctuations in the quantity and types of food they eat. This phenomenon relates to a concept called body weight "set-point." Experiments with adult humans and animals indicate that they tend to "defend" or resist changes in their "natural" body weight. Natural adult body weight is genetically determined, though it is possibly influenced by dietary habits during childhood. This weight defense mechanism is hormonal and biochemical in nature and has a primary effect on basal metabolic rate.

Basal metabolic rate, or BMR, is one of the most important factors in total body energy expenditure. It represents the energy needed to maintain the most basic bodily functions while in a totally resting state (awake, but not even digestion taking place). BMR depends on body size, so it is generally expressed as calories per unit body weight per unit time. BMR decreases with age and is generally 5 to 10 percent lower in females. For an average adult, BMR is about 1 calorie (cal) per kilogram (kg) of body weight per hour (h). Thus, for a 70 kg man (154 lb):

$$\text{BMR} = 70 \text{ kg} \times (1 \text{ cal/kg/h}) \times 24 \text{ h} = 1{,}680 \text{ cal/day}$$

BMR may vary considerably from person to person, with a 10 percent range above or below average not uncommon. Believe it or not, BMR is typically 30 to 50 percent of a person's total daily energy expenditure. It may be affected by diet and diet changes, climate, and drugs.

Body weight "set-point" experiments have shown that when a person's food intake is restricted below normal, the body rapidly becomes more efficient in using the available calories. One major way the body accomplishes this is to reduce its BMR. Likewise, in sustained overeating, the body uses food less efficiently and the BMR increases. Since BMR is such a large portion of total energy expenditure, it is clear why typical weight loss or weight gain diets have relatively small effects on body weight. Even when food intake is not modified, the typical 10 percent range found from person to person above or below average BMR values helps explain why some people can eat seemingly huge amounts of food on a regular basis without becoming overweight. Studies have also shown that when food restriction or overeating end, the body rapidly returns to its "set-point" weight. If, however, you add an exercise program to a modified food intake, you change other factors in the caloric (energy) balance equation, which help change your body weight and body composition toward more desirable levels.

When the energy needs for normal daily activities are added to the BMR needs, the average daily energy expenditure becomes approximately 35 calories per kilogram of bodyweight (15 to 16 calories per pound). So if you weigh 60 kilograms (132 pounds), you'll use about 2,100 calories a day. Athletes with busy training schedules may require more than 50 calories per kilogram of bodyweight (23 calories per pound) a day.

The energy cost for typical activities is readily available in nutrition and physiology texts, and information on the energy content of most foods can be found in cookbooks and on package labels. Using information of this type, you can calculate and compare your approximate daily energy intake and expenditure.

The table below lists the energy cost of several common activities. Using this table we can determine how long a 70-kilogram person (154 pounds) must jog (at a 12-minute-per-mile pace) or circuit weight-train to "burn off" a 250-calorie candy bar: 250 calories divided by 9 calories per minute gives 28 minutes. For those of you having difficulty gaining or losing weight, it would be revealing for you to estimate your caloric output and input daily for several weeks using the proper energy cost and food content tables.

The thought of having to exercise 28 minutes to compensate for eating a candy bar may seem discouraging, but there is much good news to the story. Regular exercise itself results in considerable cumulative energy expenditure over weeks and months. That energy—those calories—would otherwise be stored as fat or help maintain a given body fat level. In addition, exercise can maintain your metabolic rate well above normal levels for hours after an exercise period ends. This is due to physiological processes that are active to restore your body to its normal state (homeostasis) after heavy exertion. This effect can easily double the caloric cost of the exercise alone. With regular exercise, BMR may also be slightly higher than without exercise. Since BMR affects energy expenditure 24 hours a day, even a 1 to 2 percent increase could result in the burning of hundreds of extra calories each week.

Research also suggests that appetite is decreased in those who regularly exercise, compared to those who do not. Thus, although an hour of exercise may burn only a few hundred extra calories during that hour, the long-term cumulative effect will be a much greater energy expenditure than without exercise, plus a lower caloric intake and better health and physical condition.

ENERGY COST OF COMMON ACTIVITIES

Activity	Energy Cost (cal/min)*
Sleeping	1–1.5
Standing	2–2.5
Desk work	2–2.5
Slow walking (3 mph)	4–5
Cleaning windows	4–5
Golf	4–5
Painting	5–6
Cycling (8 mph)	5–6
Badmitton	5–6
Walking (4 mph)	6–7
Tennis	7–8
Snow shovelling	7–9
Circuit weight training	7–9
Jogging (12 minutes/mile)	8–10
Swimming	5–10
Handball, racquetball, squash	10–11+
Walking up stairs	10–11+
Basketball	10–11+
Skiing (alpine)	10–11+
Skiing (cross country)	12–15+

*For a 70-kg (154-pound) person.

The combination of a regular exercise program and modified but balanced diet can produce the desired changes in your body weight and/or body fat levels.

Always remember that body weight changes can occur due to changes in lean body tissue (such as muscle) and/or fat. Diet as well as exercise determines the extent of change in each type of body tissue. Your body weight may stay constant while significant improvements occur in your body composition. *If you diet without exercising, it is likely that a significant percentage of any weight lost will be muscle tissue.* This is highly undesirable and emphasizes the value of combining exercise with any diet plan. Likewise, those of you trying to gain weight need exercise to assure gains in muscle weight rather than fat alone.

When reducing your body weight with the aid of exercise, you must realize that body fat tends to be lost in reverse location order to which it was gained. In other words, if (due to genetics) fat is first increased (stored) in your abdominal area, then your buttocks, and finally your thighs, it will be lost first from your thighs and last from your abdomen. This is true even if you do a lot of abdominal exercises. You may tighten your abdomen and make it look much better, but the fat stored there decreases according to overall body fat losses and genetic storage patterns. Research indicates that so called "spot reducing" is simply not possible.

Look back at the "energy cost" table and note the high caloric cost of locomotion activities such as walking at a fast pace and climbing stairs. Any activity that requires moving the entire weight of your body uses a lot of energy, particularly if you are overweight. You can capitalize on this fact if you are trying to lose weight. Park your car at the far end of the parking lot at work, or get off the elevator a floor early and walk some stairs. This type of physical activity is particularly valuable after meals since it stimulates extra energy expenditure during digestion. Since we are seldom active in the late evening, late meals should be avoided. Having a bigger breakfast and lunch is much better since activities during the day will help burn the calories from these meals and reduce or eliminate excess energy storage as fat. Also, daily body rhythms affect metabolic rate, which is higher during the day.

PROPERTIES AND FUNCTIONS OF THE FOOD TYPES

Carbohydrates

"Carbos" should provide the majority of calories in your diet, from 50 to 60 percent. They are classified into three groups:

1. Monosaccharides or simple sugars, such as fructose and glucose (dextrose), which are found in fruits and vegetables
2. Disaccharides, such as sucrose and lactose, which are found in fruits and vegetables or milk, respectively, are combinations of two monosaccharides, and are easily digested
3. Polysaccharides, such as starch (as found in potatoes and pasta), cellulose, and glycogen (the storage form of glucose)

There is no dietary requirement for carbos since, if need be, they are easily synthesized from proteins and the glycerol component of triglycerides, a type of fat. Excess intake results in storage in muscle and the liver as glycogen, or conversion and storage as triglycerides.

Glucose, blood sugar, is the preferred energy source for exercising and is the primary energy source used by the central nervous system. When muscle or liver glycogen stores are reduced, through energy use during activity, fats are likely to become the preferred energy source. One adaptation to extensive endurance training is a more rapid shift to fat metabolism during exercise; this is called the "glycogen sparing effect." Several of the B vitamins are very important for proper carbohydrate metabolism, and the need for them increases as energy expenditure increases.

Ingestion of high carbohydrate (simple sugar) foods such as honey and candy just prior to physical activity is not beneficial. Absorption is slow from the stomach, and the sudden rise in blood sugar causes a rapid release of insulin, which reduces blood sugar.

You should try to keep the glycogen stores in your muscles and liver at high levels if you're going to be doing prolonged exercise of any kind. One way is to combine regular endurance exercise with either a balanced diet or a slightly carbo-rich diet. It is thought that a constant very high carbohydrate diet may impede the glycogen sparing effect by reducing fat metabolism. This is undesirable since fat stores have much greater potential for providing a prolonged energy supply than do liver and muscle glycogen stores.

For some special situations, such as running a marathon or competing in a triathalon, glycogen stores may be temporarily elevated to unusually high levels by a technique called "glycogen supercompensation" or "carbo loading." This method involves an exhaustive exercise session to lower glycogen stores five to seven days before the "event," followed by two or three days on a high-fat, high-protein diet with very little carbohydrate. This is then followed by three or four days on a high-carbohydrate diet. The effect of this procedure is to more than double normal levels of stored glycogen. However, some people react poorly to such extreme diet changes, and the method should be used only a few times in a year, if at all.

A less drastic "loading" technique is to go directly to a very high carbo diet after the exhaustive exercise session. This method will probably increase glycogen stores to one-and-a-half times their normal level.

It is generally accepted that the above techniques are worthwhile only for endurance events lasting longer than one hour.

Fats

Because of its high caloric value of 9 calories per gram, fat is the most important and efficient way for the body to store energy. Fat also is an important insulating material for the body and it protects various internal organs. A balanced diet should generally have about 30 percent of the total caloric content in the form of fats, although wide variations in the amount of dietary fat seem to be compatible with good health. You won't be surprised to hear that a high fat diet is particularly undesirable if you're trying to maintain or lose body fat. This is because fat has a high caloric content and our bodies are metabolically energy efficient in converting dietary fat to body fat. Fats carry flavors making foods more palatable and take longer to digest, giving satiety value to a meal. There is no specific requirement for fat as a nutrient, since it can be synthesized from excess carbohydrates and protein in the diet. However, there are a few "essential" fatty acids, such as linoleic acid found in vegetable oils, which must be consumed regularly.

Fats, or lipids, can be classified in several ways. Fatty acid "chains" are common and exist in saturated, unsaturated, and polyunsaturated forms. Saturated fatty acids are typical of animal fats and are usually solid at room temperature. Unsaturated fatty acids are usually of vegetable origin and liquid at room temperature. Exceptions include chicken fat (unsaturated), fish oils (polyunsaturated), and coconut oil (saturated).

Triglycerides (TG) are a very common form of fat. Dietary fats consist mostly of TG, as does stored body fat. TGs are composed of three fatty acid chains joined to a glycerol molecule. Fatty acids cannot be converted to carbohydrate (such as glucose) but glycerol can. TGs have been implicated in coronary heart disease, but there is no proof of a cause-and-effect relationship. Diets high in saturated fats are more likely to raise blood lipid (fat) levels than those containing mostly unsaturated fats. A proper diet combined with regular exercise has been shown to be effective in lowering blood lipids.

Glycerol, fatty acids, and other molecules join to form additional biological structures, such as phosphoglycerides, which are important components of biological membranes. Lecithin, found in "organ meats" like heart and liver, is another common member of this group and is important in fat digestion and metabolism.

Steroids, such as androgens, estrogens, and cholesterol, form another group of lipids. Cholesterol is essential for the formation of adrenal and gonadal hormones, as well as other important body compounds. It can be synthesized by the body from carbohydrates and fats in the diet. Cholesterol levels in the blood have been related to atherosclerosis in a statistical manner, but—again —a cause-and-effect relationship has not been established. Exercise and lower consumption of saturated fat appear to be effective in reducing this coronary risk factor.

Lipids may also combine with proteins (lipoproteins) and sugars and are frequently transported in the blood via such compounds. Lipoproteins are found in a range of densities (very low to very high) and their relative concentration in the blood has also been related to atherosclerosis. A large proportion of high density lipoproteins (HDL) to low density lipoproteins (LDL) is considered desirable for good health. Weight training and other forms of exercise have the beneficial effect of increasing HDL/LDL ratios.

Protein

Protein is generally considered the most important nutrient for our bodies. Proteins are large molecules composed of amino acids. Nine of approximately 20 known amino acids are essential; that is, these nine *must* be supplied regularly in the diet since they cannot be synthesized by the body. Foods containing all essential amino acids are said to provide complete proteins, or to be of high biological value. Meats, fish, poultry, eggs, and dairy products provide complete proteins. If incomplete proteins are consumed in proper combination, within approximately two hours of each other, complete protein can be formed. In other words, if five essential amino acids are provided by one food and the other four by a second food, then the available protein "building blocks" are complete. The non-essential amino acids can be synthesized by our bodies if not provided by the foods we eat. This process of forming complete proteins from proper combinations of incomplete proteins is called *mutual supplementation* and is an important process for vegetarians whose meatless diets might otherwise not provide all the essential amino acids.

Its central position in the structure of body tissues makes protein such an important nutrient. Protein can be used for energy, but that occurs mainly in extreme situations when fat and carbohydrate stores are very low or exhausted, as during starvation. We hear about increased protein need most frequently as it concerns strength athletes who are trying to build or maintain a large amount of muscle tissue. Endurance athletes, however, also have significant protein needs, because of their increased use and turnover of oxidative enzymes, myoglobin, and hemoglobin, to mention just a few of the increased tissue demands. In an active person's diet, protein should probably constitute 15 to 20 percent of the calories. The recommended daily allowance (RDA) of protein for adults is 0.8 grams per Kg of body weight, or about 1 gram for every 2¾ pounds of body weight. Athletes on vigorous training programs may consume a gram or more of protein daily for each pound of body weight.

Protein supplements are probably not needed for an individual who consumes a balanced diet with the total caloric content adjusted to his or her activity level. If food consumption is erratic and unbalanced, protein, vitamin, and mineral supplements can help. All supplements should be introduced into the diet gradually, since, for example, a sudden intake of even recommended amounts of protein powder could cause digestion problems, such as diarrhea. Excess protein intake is converted to fat for storage, and nitrogen, a major component of protein, is excreted.

If you are using a protein or amino acid supplement, it is important that the amino acid content be reasonably balanced. There are specific absorption sites in the small intestine for different groups of amino acids. If a given site is responsible for absorption of amino acids 1, 2, and 3, and 1 is present in much greater concentration than 2 and 3, then very little of 2 and 3 will be used. This could have an adverse effect on protein metabolism and tissue building, especially if 2 or 3 are essential amino acids. Eating a balanced diet is one of the best ways to obtain a proper distribution of the various amino acids and make best use of them in protein metabolism.

Vitamins and Minerals

Vitamins are organic compounds important for proper functioning of the body through their biochemical involvement in regulating metabolic processes. Vitamins are subdivided into two major groups: fat soluble (A, D, E, and K), carried in fatty foods and stored within body fat; and water soluble (B complex and C). Ideally, you should be able to get all the vitamins you need by consuming a balanced diet with the needed caloric content. Cooking and processing foods, however, can reduce vitamin content. Vitamin enrichment and fortification of some foods by manufacturers helps correct this problem but doesn't necessarily solve it. A moderate potency vitamin and mineral supplement can assure you of adequate intake with little or no danger of overdose. Standard multivitamin and mineral tablets can be purchased for about $5 per hundred. A nickel a day is a small investment for assuring adequate intake, even if much of the supplement is excess and passed through the system. Many highly trained athletes take large doses of vitamin and mineral supplements, but there is no conclusive research to indicate that such large dosages improve performance. Much is yet to be learned about the positive and negative effects of "megavitamin" consumption.

It is important to remember that vitamins do *not* constitute a meal, since they have no caloric value. Also, they're best absorbed and utilized if taken in conjunction with food. Fat soluble vitamins can be harmful if taken in large quantities over a long period, because they accumulate in body fat. Vitamin and mineral needs can vary from person to person even if activity levels are equal. This may be due, in part, to genetics and the efficiency with which a person's body uses and stores vitamins and minerals. You should consider the recommended daily allowances as guidelines, but if you have doubts or concerns about your intake, check with a nutritionist or your doctor. Incidentally, there is no evidence that vitamins from "natural" sources are more effective than synthetic vitamins.

Minerals serve a variety of functions in the body. Some are used as structural components, such as calcium and phosphorus in bones and teeth. Iron is a needed component of hemoglobin in red blood cells, while other minerals are important in enzymes and hormones. Minerals also perform regulatory functions, as in muscular contraction and nerve impulse conduction. They are classified as either *major* or *trace* elements, depending on the amounts needed for proper body function. Supplements, as discussed above, may be a worthwhile, inexpensive investment, particularly if you are physically active and have an erratic diet.

Water

Water, to say the least, is a very important substance for most bodily functions. We can survive only a short time without water intake. Due to its importance in temperature regulation, water needs for active people and those in hot climates are considerably increased and must be satisfied. At the very minimum, you should drink several glasses a day, especially if you are exercising regularly. The human thirst mechanisms are weak, so although your thirst may feel quenched, you are still likely to be somewhat dehydrated from normal. Always try to drink some fluid at regular intervals during exercise. Smaller amounts (5 to 8 ounces) of cold liquid taken frequently are better than isolated large intakes. Water is the best liquid for avoiding dehydration. There are many commercially available drinks designed to replace minerals, as well as fluid, and to provide simple sugars for energy, but these are too concentrated to be absorbed rapidly and should be diluted with water before use. Salt tablets are definitely not needed, since sodium and other mineral losses are rapidly replaced with normal meals.

ERGOGENIC AIDS

"Ergogenic" comes from the Greek *ergon,* meaning work, and *genic,* which means producing. Ergogenic aids are substances and/or procedures that may tend to increase work capacity or physical performance level. They range from such familiar substances as caffeine, alcohol, vitamin, mineral, and protein

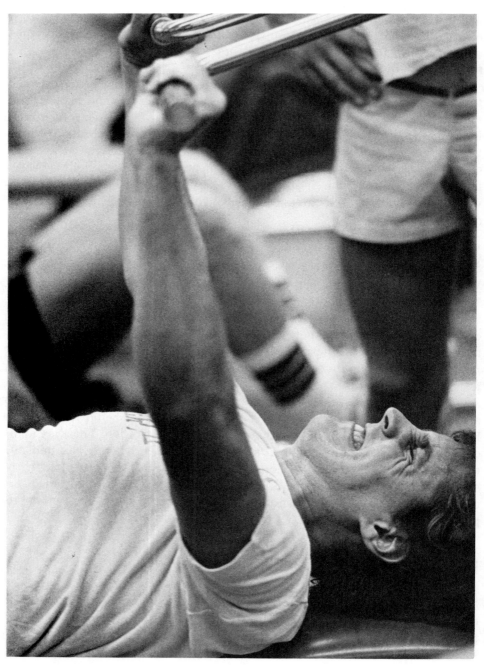

Good strength training is a product of hard work, sensible nutrition and a complete and simple program. Stay away from dangerous ergogenic aids such as amphetamines and steroids.

supplements, and pure oxygen to prescription drugs, such as amphetamines and
anabolic steroids. Common ergogenic procedures used to improve performance
are mental imagery, biofeedback, hypnosis, and massage.

It is impossible to discuss adequately every type of ergogenic aid in a book
of this scope. However, those interested in incorporating any of them into their
strength regimen should be warned: certain ergogenic aids, such as amphetamines—a type of stimulant—and anabolic steroids—drugs that increase muscle
bulk—are known to have dangerous, and in some cases, irreversible side effects.
With amphetamines, these can include psychological dependence, excessive
use, and the risk of fatal overdosing; with anabolic steroids, permanent growth
stoppage in children and teens, irreversible masculinization in women, and high
blood pressure, liver abnormalities, and testicular atrophy in men. (In addition,
high blood pressure and liver abnormalities can occur in the other two groups
mentioned.) Both amphetamines and anabolic steroids are currently banned in
most athletic circles throughout the world, and certainly have no place in an
average person's training program. *Stay away from these drugs,* and when
considering ergogenic aids of any kind, be sure that first you know exactly what
their effects, risks, and dangers are.

Muscle Stimulation

Electrical muscle stimulation (EMS) is a procedure that can be classified as an
ergogenic aid. It involves external stimulation of muscle fibers by applying
electrical voltages to the skin surface over the fibers. Parameters such as voltage
level, stimulation frequency, and rest intervals between stimulations must be
chosen carefully to improve muscle strength, endurance, and size. Such techniques
have been used successfully for years in rehabilitation work, but the Soviet Union
has been a leader in their application to conditioning athletes.

You must realize, however, that EMS itself is not exercise. Some elite athletes
have occasionally used it in conjunction with the numerous other components of
their overall training program, but no one would ever use it alone as a means of
conditioning the body. Even in rehabilitation work, it is generally used with other
treatments and exercises. EMS does not burn calories to any appreciable degree and
does not remove fat. Much remains to be learned about the benefits and limitations
of this training aid.

Running,
Stretching
and Lifting - If you
dare to be great

7

Training Methods for the "Serious" Athlete

In Chapter 5 you saw examples of several types of weight training programs and many techniques for adding variety to them. Among the programs I showed you was a typical strength training cycle, whose phases progressed from higher to lower repetitions per set. You'll remember that the high-rep phase of the cycle had certain purposes and goals, such as reducing body fat and building muscle tissue, whose attainment was important for success in the subsequent phases where one purpose was building strength. This concept of one phase of a training cycle "potentiating" the body for increased adaptation in the next phase is at the heart of a training technique called *periodization*, which is used in one form or another by most world-class athletes.

So far in this book we've studied strength training as a form of exercise in and of itself, although the basic concepts and training principles presented can, and should, be applied to all exercise programs. However, when you employ a training program not only for strength and general fitness but also for improved performance in a particular sport or physical activity, you need to consider some additional factors.

First, you should realize that the emphasis of

189

Most serious athletes vary their strength training cycles for maximum performance during competition.

your overall training program, not just the strength component, should change during different times of the year. No one can effectively train for strength, power, endurance, and sport techniques at the same time. Thus, during different periods you should emphasize developing different physical (and psychological) requirements for effective participation in your sport, while trying to maintain or minimize the loss of other requirements. Many athletes, for example, find it works best for them to concentrate mainly on strength development during the off-season and pre-season months, and then to try to maintain their strength level while concentrating on applying it effectively to their particular sport. This is easier to do if the chosen strength training exercises work the various muscle groups of the body in movement patterns that are similar to those occurring in the actual sport (that is, the specificity of training principle).

Second, the most productive way to develop the various components of fitness, and the motor skills (sport technique) needed for specific sports or types of physical activity, is to train in cycles. Each cycle, or period of weeks or months, has a major goal and one or more minor goals. Planning such training programs, with the end goal being the best possible overall condition for a given activity during a given period of time, is called *periodization of training*.

For some athletes, cyclic training makes obvious good sense. Track-and-field athletes, gymnasts, boxers, and weightlifters, for example, have only a few really important contests per year. For these types of athletes, training cycles can easily be designed to lead up to a "big event" and put the competitor in top shape for his or her sport.

The following is an example of this type of situation. It's a program designed for a female gymnast who competes in the "all-around," which consists of four events. Later, we'll look at some useful ways to train in cycles for seasonal sports, such as skiing and football, and year-round sports such as racquetball and squash.

BASICS OF A TRAINING CYCLE FOR GYMNASTICS

The multi-event nature of the all-around in women's gymnastics requires considerable stamina to maintain performance at the highest level throughout prolonged competitions. The individual events themselves require great strength, power, flexibility, and movement skills. For this example, let's consider an athlete who has just finished several weeks of rest, relaxation, and low-level recreational activities following her competitive year. She now has three months available to prepare for the first meet of the new competitive year. What should she do?

Rather than trying to develop and improve all of the above-mentioned components of competitive readiness simultaneously, her coach designs a training plan in cyclic form. The first cycle of her "new year" plan will last three months, the time available until the first meet of the year.

Three phases are generally contained in a training cycle, due to properties of Selye's General Adaptation Syndrome, which we discussed in Chapter 5. The first training phase takes into account the *alarm reaction* of GAS and gets the body accustomed, or reaccustomed, to strenuous physical activity. The remainder of the first phase and the second phase of the training cycle take into account the *resistance phase* of GAS, which is a time when the body adapts to the program and increases its potential for a quality performance in the sport it's being conditioned for. This middle phase of a training cycle is called the *preparatory phase*. The third phase may be called a *pre-competition* or *competition phase* of the cycle, when total workload (volume of training) is cut back to permit the body to recover completely from the first two phases, and to allow extra attention for fine points of technique. For simplicity in this example, let's assume each phase of the cycle lasts four weeks.

Phase One

Given the nature of gymnastics and the demands of competing in the all-around, the major emphasis of phase one would probably be to develop stamina, cardiovascular fitness, and good overall physical condition. Of lesser importance for this first phase is the development of strength, flexibility, and technique for the competitive events. Thus, the initial training phase would emphasize running (both longer distances and shorter repetitive intervals) or cycling, basketball, circuit weight workouts (using higher reps per set and short rest intervals), or other more or less continuous low intensity activities. Actual gymnastics practice would likely occupy less than one-third of the athlete's weekly training time.

Phase Two

Phase two of this cycle should probably emphasize strength and power development, although flexibility and gymnastics technique take on increased importance, too. The gymnast should maintain her basic fitness and stamina level (improved in Phase One) by following a well-planned, strenuous program involving and stressing the components just mentioned. Three weight workouts each week, with a good choice of primary and assistance exercises, should provide her with the needed strength and power improvement. Her flexibility can be developed during warm-up and on in-between days when she practices gymnastics technique. Light technique work can also be done on weight training days.

Phase Three

Now that the gymnast is stronger and has good stamina and flexibility, she can concentrate on perfecting her technique in the competitive events during phase three of the training cycle. She can maintain strength and power with just two weight workouts each week. Stamina and general fitness are maintained simply by her participation in the long daily workouts during which she repeatedly practices parts of her competitive routines.

The illustration graphically depicts the emphasis of major training goal components during the total three-month cycle. Note the special alterations that occur the week before the meet; namely, she works almost exclusively on her gymnastic techniques, while other components are essentially eliminated from the program.

Each week during this three-month cycle is planned ahead by her coach and should include a lot of variation. The days of each week are also planned ahead, using some of the ideas we discussed in Chapter 5. Stamina and technique work are varied day to day and week to week in a manner similar to the strength training variations. If the details of the program are properly planned and followed, the athlete will be "peaked" for a quality performance.

Emphasis During a Gymnastics Training Cycle

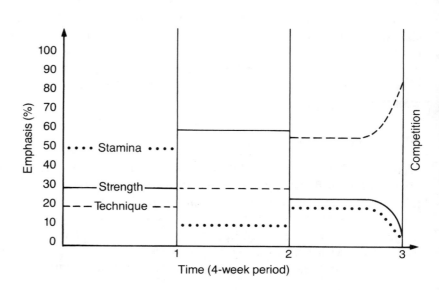

The above example was presented in very general form to illustrate the typical considerations used to construct a training cycle. Depending on the needs and experience of a given athlete, the amount of time available for training, and so on, different priorities could receive emphasis at different times, or for different durations during a given cycle.

TRAINING FOR TEAM AND SEASONAL SPORTS

If your interest is in team sports such as baseball, basketball, and football, or seasonal sports such as skiing, you can also benefit from a planned training cycle. With any of these sports or similar seasonal activities, an intelligent approach is to use pre-season, in-season, and post-season cycles. In this kind of a program you condition yourself not for a few major competitions each year, as in the previous example, but for a period of weeks or months when games or participation is frequent.

Most pre-season cycles initially emphasize the development of stamina, muscular endurance, and cardiovascular fitness. A later phase of this cycle could be designed to improve strength and motor skills (technique) involved in the sport or activity itself.

The in-season cycle generally involves a cutback in most components of training due to the time and energy you spend participating in the actual sport or activity. Regular and frequent competition or participation should, by itself, minimize loss of stamina and endurance and enhance motor skills. Strength maintenance, or minimizing strength loss, can be accomplished with one or two weight workouts each week.

The post-season cycle is a good time for you to emphasize strength development, with relatively little of your total training time devoted to other goals.

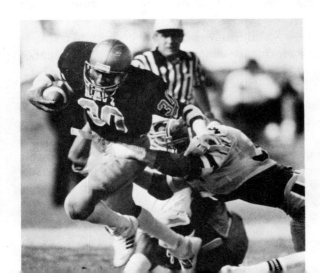

Football players generally follow pre-season, in-season, and post-season strength training cycles.

A weight training cycle similar to the one I presented at the end of Chapter 5 would fit well into this cycle of training.

TRAINING FOR YEAR-ROUND ACTIVITIES

You may wonder how to plan cyclic training for an activity like tennis or racquetball, which you can play all year long. The answer is simply to plan training cycles as you would for a seasonal sport. Emphasize certain components of fitness in different cycles, and accept the fact that during some cycles you will not be playing at your best. In the long run, however, your physical abilities will increase more than with a non-varying, non-cyclic program, and you will eventually play closer to your genetic potential.

One of the greatest mistakes some competitive weightlifters make in their year-long training programs is to always train with low reps and heavy weights. They seem to have a psychological need to handle "big" weights and feel very strong all the time. Their eagerness for ever-increasing personal lifting records prevents them from devoting the emphasis of a single phase in a training cycle to basic conditioning, flexibility, or technique work. Such athletes may never reach their true physical potential.

GUIDELINES FOR PLANNING A TRAINING CYCLE

When you begin a period of training, your performance capabilities usually decrease in the first week or two. This is because your body is experiencing the *alarm stage* of the General Adaptation Syndrome; it needs to get used to or readapt to the demands of exercise. You can minimize this decline in performance, and accompanying muscle soreness, by gradually working into the new training program.

This stage is followed by a period during which your body is adapting to the exercise stressors and your performance capabilities increase. This is called the *preparatory phase* of training, since your body is being "prepared" for higher performance.

If the exercise stressors are too great or last too long, your body may go into an *exhaustion stage* where performance capability decreases and you are said to be *overtrained*. With proper planning, you can avoid overtraining and maintain an elevated performance level for a relatively long period, preferably when competitions are occurring or when you are participating frequently in your activity.

After this so-called *competition phase,* you should cut back your training so your body can make a smooth transition into another "prep" phase without getting overtrained. This transition phase permits your body to recuperate fully from the stress of training and competition so that it can successfully adapt to new exercise stressors.

A complete training cycle consisting of a readaptation (or transition) phase, a prep phase, and a contest phase is often called a *macrocycle.*

How Long Should Each Phase Last?

Typical time periods for the different phases of a training cycle look like this:

1. Readaptation or transition phase: one to two weeks
2. Preparatory phase: four to eight weeks
3. Contest phase: three to six weeks

These are certainly flexible within reasonable limits and depend on the sport you are training for. As you become more "experienced," the phases may tend to last longer, but you must discover for yourself what works best for you and adjust the phase durations accordingly.

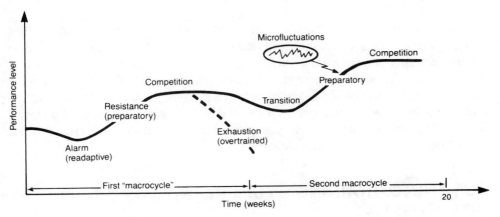

Training-cycle analogy to GAS

How Do Load, Volume, and Intensity Change for Each Phase?

For the *strength training component* of a program, each phase of a cycle can be characterized by relative values for load, intensity, and volume.

1. Readaptation or transition phase: low load, intensity, and volume
2. Preparatory phase: moderate to high load, intensity, and volume
3. Contest phase: low to moderate load, high intensity, low volume

Earlier, I mentioned that other sports, like running, also have *objective measures* for the *volume* and *intensity* of training. This is also important for you to consider—in addition to load, volume, and intensity values for the strength training component of your program—when planning the weeks that make up your training cycle. In a prep phase, for example, there should be "microfluctuations" day to day in the volume and intensity of *total* training. If you use a light strength training day to go heavy in some other component of your program (for example, practicing technique in the high jump), then that day is a heavy training day *overall*. This cannot occur continuously or over-training will result; your body must have light *overall* training days to help it recuperate totally from heavy ones. Your performance capabilities gradually increase during most of a training cycle, but they are lowered immediately after heavy training sessions. The fact that a prep phase is characterized by moderate to high load and intensity does not mean that periodic daily reductions cannot occur. These reductions result in overall light training days, which generally have a large volume reduction but smaller intensity decrease relative to the heavy days.

The idea of repeated "macrocycles" is to raise performance capabilities "step by step." One complete cycle may emphasize developing a particular component that is important to your sport—say, strength or technique—or it may be more general in nature. As your most important competitions or activities approach, you should be as ready as possible for a maximum performance. To show how volume measures (total reps for weight lifting, total distance for running, and so on) can help you plan phases of a training cycle, consider the situation of a competitive weightlifter.

ADVANCED TRAINING CYCLE PLANNING FOR WEIGHTLIFTING

From past experience, an Olympic-style weightlifting coach determines that the coming training year for his lifter should contain a total lifting volume of 10,000 reps. The first six months of the year contain about 55 percent of the volume, since, on average, training during the first half of the year is done with slightly lower weights and slightly higher reps. This leaves 4,500 reps (45 percent) for the second six months of the athlete's training year, which concludes with the competition of greatest importance, the National Championship.

The training year is divided into 12 four-week periods, with four weeks of the year set aside for vacation and active rest. Thus, six training periods are contained in the second half of the year. The volume for this half of the year, 4,500 reps, is divided *unequally* among the six periods so as to vary the exercise stressors imposed on the athlete. There are many ways to proportion the 4,500 reps, and one reasonable scheme is to have a 700, 1,100, 600, 900, 700, and 500 rep period. Obviously, the training volume should decrease before the major competition, and the sample scheme above has only 1,200 of the 4,500 reps in the last two of six four-week periods. Also, right after the heaviest period (1,100 reps), volume is decreased by almost 50 percent, to 600 reps. Such a decrease is often planned so that the athlete can successfully participate in a competition of lesser importance at the end of this low volume period.

Once the coach decides on the division of lifting volume among the available training periods, he must divide each period's volume *unequally* among its four weeks, to have variation in the program. If he considers the 900 rep period of this example, a reasonable division would be 200, 250, 150, 300 reps per week. This provides for one light, one heavy, and two medium volume weeks. The first week in the following period would be light to moderate in volume since the last week of this period is heavy (300 reps). The coach uses common sense, experience, and training literature to help determine this weekly division of volume.

The coach must also subdivide each week's volume among the planned training days. A division of 55, 40, 75, 30 reps per day would be reasonable for the first week (200 total reps). Four training days in this week were chosen because 200 reps fit well into this number of days. If an advanced lifter were to have 400 reps scheduled for a heavy week, five days would probably be used. If a very large volume were assigned to a single day (125 reps), two training sessions rather than one might be used on that day.

Finally, the exercises, sets, and reps for each day must be chosen. Methods for doing this were discussed in Chapter 5. Light days would have two or three core exercises, while heavy days might have four to six. The sets per exercise usually range from three to six (plus warm-up sets). Assistance exercises follow core exercises and may involve only one or two sets.

The coach makes these types of subdivisions for each four-week period of the year, resulting in a day-by-day training plan for the entire year. He may have to make modifications during the year, due to unexpected progress or lack of it by the athlete, but these should be minor if the coach is experienced and has really thought out the program relative to the athlete's needs and abilities. If injury or illness occurs, it must be overcome and training must be adapted with as little change as possible. The coach must also fit "active rest" (such as

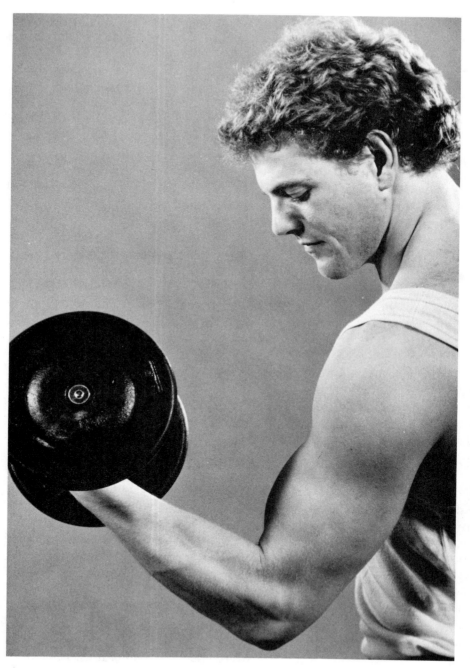

Learn your body's limits to avoid overtraining. Good luck, and be strong!

running, cycling, or basketball) into the program on non-training days, to build or maintain stamina and cardiovascular fitness without interfering with the primary training goals.

This example of how to use training volume division in the planning of a long-term training cycle can be applied to many situations. If running or swimming, for example, is included in your total training program, then the distance covered is the volume measure, as stated in Chapter 5. You can divide this training volume unequally day to day, week to week, and month to month, just as you would the number of reps in your strength training exercises. Likewise, you can consider the time spent in the actual practice of your sport as a volume measure, and can divide it in a reasonable way, day by day and week by week, within the phases of your training cycles. Periodization is an extremely valuable tool that is universally used in high-level training. Its success depends on how well you apply the basic training principles we've discussed to your program, how well you learn about your body's responses to different training programs, and, to some extent, how you use your imagination.

CONCLUSION

There are many ways to develop the various components of total body fitness. In this book I've shown you how all components can be developed using a properly designed strength training program with or without additional modes of exercise. The key step in designing a successful exercise program is to decide which components of fitness you need to emphasize, without neglecting the others, and then to plan how to develop these components with appropriate techniques—not necessarily the most advanced.

I have emphasized strength fitness in this book and have explained very basic to advanced training methods. For most of you, if you start using the simpler techniques you'll make good progress initially and be able to continue making progress for a long time by gradually adding advanced training methods to your program.

Remember: It's not where you start in terms of fitness that's important. Rather, it's that you make progress toward better fitness. Don't spend a lot of time comparing yourself with others; compare yourself with where you were a few weeks or months earlier—it's *your* progress that's important. Train hard and on a regular schedule, but don't overtrain—remember the value of light training days. And finally, watch what you eat; nutrition is an important contributing factor to the success of any exercise program. Good luck!

Resources

For information on Olympic-style weightlifting, contact:

> The U. S. Weightlifting Federation (USWF)
> U.S. Olympic Complex
> 1750 E. Boulder St.,
> Colorado Springs, CO 80909

For information on powerlifting, contact:

> Powerlifting U.S.A.
> P. O. Box 467
> Camarillo, CA 93011

For information on bodybuilding, contact:

> The International Federation of Body Builders (IFBB)
> c/o Wieder Enterprises
> 21100 Erwin St.
> Woodland Hills, CA 91367

For information on strength training and conditioning programs for sports, contact:

> The National Strength Conditioning Association (NSCA)
> P. O. Box 81410
> Lincoln, NE 68501

For more general information on weight training and associated topics and products, check your local magazine counters for monthly or bimonthly publications such as *Muscle and Fitness, Strength and Health, Sports Fitness,* and *Shape* magazines.

Further Readings

Chapter 1

Astrand, P., and K. Rodahl. *Textbook of Work Physiology—Physiological Bases of Exercise,* 2nd edition. New York: McGraw Hill, 1977.

Caiozzo, V. J., J. J. Perrine, and V. R. Edgerton. "Alterations in the In Vivo Force-Velocity Relationship." *Medicine and Science in Sports and Exercise.* Vol. 12, No. 2 (1980, abstract), p. 134; *Journal of Applied Physiology.* Vol. 51, No. 3 (1981), pp. 750–754.

Coyle, E. F., and D. Feiring. "Muscular Power Improvements: Specificity of Training Velocity." *Medicine and Science in Sports and Exercise.* Vol. 12, No. 2 (1980, abstract), p. 134.

Darcus, H. D. "Discussion on an Evaluation of the Methods of Increasing Muscle Strength." *Proceedings of the Royal Society of Medicine.* Vol. 49 (December 1956), pp. 999–1006.

Edington, D. W., and V. R. Edgerton. *The Biology of Physical Activity.* Boston: Houghton Mifflin, 1976.

Gardner, G. W. "Specificity of Strength Changes of the Exercised and Nonexercised Limb Following Isometric Training." *Research Quarterly.* Vol. 34, No. 1 (1963), pp. 98–101.

Hayes, R. C. "A Theory of the Mechanisms of Muscular Strength Development Based upon EMG Evidence of Motor Unit Synchronization." *Biomechanics of Sports and Kinanthropometry* (F. Landry and W. Organ, eds.). Miami: Symposium Specialists, 1978, pp. 69–77.

Hakkinen, K. and P. V. Komi. "Electromyographic Changes During Strength Training and Detraining." *Medicine and Science in Sports and Exercise.* Vol. 15, No. 6 (1983), pp. 455–460.

Komi, P. V. "Neuromuscular Performance: Factors Influencing Force and Speed Production." *Scandinavian Journal of Sports Science.* Vol. 1, No. 1 (1979), pp. 2–15.

Lamb. D. R. *Physiology of Exercise: Responses and Adaptations.* New York: Macmillan, 1978.

Milner-Brown, H. S., R. B. Stein, and R. G. Lee. "Synchronization of Human Motor Units: Possible Roles of Exercise and Supraspinal Reflexes." *Electroencephalograph and Clinical Neurophysiology.* Vol. 38 (1975), pp. 245–254.

Moffroid, M., and R. H. Whipple. "Specificity of Speed of Exercise." *Physical Therapy.* Vol. 50 (1970), pp. 1693–1699.

Rasch, P. J., and R. K. Burke. *Kinesiology and Applied Anatomy,* 6th edition. Philadelphia: Lea & Febiger, 1978.

Sale, D., and D. MacDougall. "Specificity in Strength Training; A Review for the Coach and Athlete." *Sports—Science Periodical on Research and Technology in Sport* (Canada), March 1981.

Stone, M. H., D. Wilson, R. Rozenek, and H. Newton. "Anaerobic Capacity—Physiological Basis." *National Strength and Conditioning Association Journal.* Vol. 5, No. 6 (1983), pp. 40, 63–65.

Vander, A. J., J. H. Sherman, and D. S. Luciano. *Human Physiology—The Mechanisms of Body Function,* 2nd ed. New York: McGraw Hill, 1976.

Chapter 2

Anderson, B. *Stretching.* P. O. Box 2734, Fullerton, CA 92633. 1975.

Gettman, L. R., and M. L. Pollock. "Circuit Weight Training: A Critical Review of Its Physiological Benefits." *The Physician and Sports Medicine.* Vol. 9, No. 1 (January 1981), pp. 44–60.

Gettman, L. R., P. Ward, and R. D. Hagan. "Strength and Endurance Changes Through Circuit Weight Training." *National Strength & Conditioning Association Journal.* Vol. 3, No. 4 (1981), pp. 12–14.

Stone, M. H., D. P. Smith, M. Rush, and D. Carter. "Olympic Weight Lifting: Metabolic Consequences of a Workout." *Science in Weightlifting* (J. Terauds, ed.). Del Mar, CA: Academic Publishers, 1979, pp. 55–67.

Wilmore, J. H., et. al. "Physiological Alterations Consequent to Circuit Weight Training." *Medicine and Science in Sports.* Vol. 10, No. 2 (1978), pp. 79–84.

Chapter 3

Garhammer, J. "Equipment for the Development of Athletic Strength and Power." *National Strength and Conditioning Association Journal.* Vol. 3, No. 6 (December 1981), pp. 24–26.

Garhammer, J. "Turn Your Home Into a Fitness Center." *Shape.* Vol. 2, No. 4 (December 1982), pp. 68–73.

Soper, W. "Pumping Iron with Archimedes." *Technology Illustrated.* April 1983, pp. 39–41.

Starr, B. *The Strongest Shall Survive . . . Strength Training for Football.* Annapolis, MD: Fitness Products Ltd., 1976.

Stone, M. H. "Considerations in Gaining a Strength-Power Training Effect: Machines Versus Free Weights." *National Strength and Conditioning Association Journal.* Vol. 4, No. 1 (1982), pp. 22–24.

Turner, G. "More About Free Weights Versus Machines." *Muscle.* Vol. 40, No. 7 (July 1979), pp. 20–21.

Chapter 4

Algra, B. "An In-Depth Analysis of the Bench Press." *National Strength and Conditioning Association Journal.* Vol. 4, No. 5 (1982), pp. 6–7, 10–11, 70–72.

Dostal, G. "Partner Resistance Training for the Neck." *National Strength and Conditioning Association Journal.* Vol. 5, No. 3 (1983), pp. 40–44.

Garhammer, J., and H. Newton. "Bridging the Gap: Power Clean." *National Strength and Conditioning Association Journal.* Vol. 6, No. 3 (1984), pp. 40–41, 61–66.

Roundtable discussion: "The Squat and Its Application to Athletic Performance." *National Strength and Conditioning Association Journal.* Vol. 6, No. 3 (1984), pp. 10–22, 68.

Pearl, B. *Keys to the Inner Universe.* Physical Fitness Architects, P.O. Box 1080, Phoenix, OR 97535. (NOTE: This book is primarily for bodybuilders, but it contains descriptions and illustrations of almost all strength training exercises known.)

Chapter 5

Berger, R. "Effect of Varied Weight Training Programs on Strength." *Research Quarterly.* Vol. 33 (1962), pp. 168–181.

Clarke, D. H. "Adaptations in Strength and Muscular Endurance Resulting from Exercise." *Exercise and Sport Science Reviews.* Vol. 1 (1973), pp. 73–102.

Hickson, R. C. "Interference of Strength Development by Simultaneously Training for Strength and Endurance." *European Journal of Applied Physiology.* Vol. 45 (1980), pp. 255–263.

O'Shea, J. P. "Effects of Selected Weight Training Programs on the Development of Strength and Muscle Hypertrophy." *Research Quarterly.* Vol. 37 (1966), pp. 95–102.

O'Shea, J. P. *Scientific Principles and Methods of Strength Fitness,* 2nd ed. Addison-Wesley, 1976.

Seyle, H. *Stress Without Distress.* New York: J. B. Lippincott, 1974.

Selye, H. *The Stress of Life* (rev. ed., 1976; paperback ed., 1978). New York: McGraw-Hill.

Stone, M. H., H. Bryant, J. Garhammer, J. McMillan, and R. Rozenek. "A Theoretical Model of Strength Training." *National Strength and Conditioning Association Journal.* Vol. 4, No. 4 (1982), pp. 36–39.

Stowers, T., et. al. "The Short-Term Effects of Three Different Strength-Power Training Methods." *National Strength and Conditioning Association Journal.* Vol. 5, No. 3 (1983), pp. 24–27.

Yessis, M. "The Key to Strength Development: Variety." *National Strength and Conditioning Association Journal.* Vol. 3, No. 3 (1981), pp. 32–34.

Chapter 6

Alfin-Slater, R., and L. Aftergood, *Nutrition for Today.* Dubuque, IA: William C. Brown, 1973.

Allen, D. W., and B. M. Quigley. "The Role of Physical Activity in the Control of Obesity." *The Medical Journal of Australia.* September 1977, pp. 434–438.

Brownell, K. D., and A. J. Stunkard. "Physical Activity in the Development and Control of Obesity." *Obesity* (A. J. Stunkard, ed.). Philadelphia: W. B. Saunders, 1980.

"Caffeine." *Consumer Reports.* Vol. 46, No. 10 (October 1981), pp. 595–599.

Garhammer, J. "An Introduction to the Use of Electrical Muscle Stimulation with Athletes." *National Strength and Conditioning Association Journal.* Vol. 5, No. 4 (1983), pp. 44–45.

Keesey, R. E. "A Set-Point Analysis of the Regulation of Body Weight." *Obesity* (A. J. Stunkard, ed.). Philadelphia: W. B. Saunders, 1980.

O'Shea, J. P. "Anabolic Steroids in Sport: A Biophysical Evaluation." *Nutrition Reports International.* Vol. 17, No. 6 (1978), pp. 607–627.

Pennington, J. A. T., and H. N. Church. *Food Values of Portions Commonly Used,* 14th ed. New York: Harper & Row, 1985.

Roundtable discussion: "Anabolic Steroids." *National Strength and Conditioning Association Journal.* Vol. 5, No. 4 (1983), pp. 12–22.

Rozenek, R., and M. H. Stone. "Protein Metabolism Related to Athletics." *National Strength and Conditioning Association Journal.* Vol. 6, No. 2 (1984), pp. 42–45.

Stone, M. H., et. al. "Physiological Effects of a Short Term Resistive Training Program on Middle Age Untrained Men." *National Strength and Conditioning Association Journal.* Vol. 4, No. 5 (1982), pp. 16–20.

Taylor, W. N. *Anabolic Steroids and the Athlete.* Jefferson, NC: McFarland & Co., 1982.

Tran, Z. V., et. al. "The Effects of Exercise on Blood Lipids and Lipoproteins: A Meta-Analysis of Studies." *Medicine and Science in Sports and Exercise.* Vol. 15, No. 5 (1983), pp. 393–402.

U. S. Department of Agriculture. "Nutritive Value of Foods," *Home and Garden Bulletin* No. 72 (Washington, D.C.: 1977, revised).

Wright, J. *Anabolic Steroids and Sports,* Volumes I (1978) and II (1982). Sports Science Consultants, P.O. Box 633, Natick, MA 01760.

Wright, J., and M.H. Stone. "Literature Review of Research and Studies on Anabolic Steroids." *National Strength and Conditioning Association Journal.* Vol. 7, No. 5 (1985), pp 45–59.

Chapter 7

Garhammer, J. "Periodization of Strength Training for Athletes." *Track Technique.* Vol. 75 (Spring 1979), pp. 2398–2399.

Yessis, M. "The Soviet Sports Training System; The Yearly Cycle." *National Strength and Conditioning Association Journal.* Vol. 3, No. 6 (1981), pp. 20–22.

Yessis, M. "The Role of All-Round, General Physical Preparation in the Multiyear and Yearly Training Program." *National Strength and Conditioning Association Journal.* Vol. 4, No. 5 (1982), pp. 48–50.

Yessis, M. "The Role of Specialized Training in Multiyear and Yearly Training Programs." *National Strength and Conditioning Association Journal.* Vol. 4, No. 6 (1982), pp. 10–11.

Yessis, M. "The Competitive Period in the Multiyear and Yearly Training Program." *National Strength and Conditioning Association Journal.* Vol. 5, No. 1 (1983), pp. 45–46.